2002

To M

0

MW01698067

Flora Dodd

Journal of a Living Lady

Jer. 33:3

Nancy White Kelly

Flora,
You have been such a blessing to me and my family through all these years.
We'll "catch up" in heaven one of these days. Hugs,
Nancy W. Kelly

15

Journal of a Living Lady

Library of Congress Card Number: 2001116518

Kelly, Nancy White

Journal of a Living Lady: a series of up-beat newspaper columns, written by a terminally-ill cancer patient. These journals were originally published in the Sentinel Newspapers.

Medical information included in this book should not be construed as recommendations by the author or publisher. Cancer patients should be under the care of a personal physician.

All of the illustrations in this book are true to life. A few names and locations have been changed to protect privacy.

Publisher's Cataloging-in-Publication
(Provided by Quality Books, Inc.)

Kelly, Nancy White.
Journal of a living lady / Nancy White Kelly.-- 1st ed.
p. cm.
ISBN 0-9708502-04

1. Kelly, Nancy White--Health. 2. Cancer--Humor.
3. Breast--Cancer--Patients--Georgia--Biography.
4. Journalists--Georgia--Biography. I. Title.

RC280.B8K45 2001 362. 1'9699449'0092
QBI21-1 10

Printed in the U.S.A.
Morris Publishing
3212 East Highway 30
Kearney, NE 68847
1-800-650-7888

Journal of a Living Lady

It was near midnight, the 23rd of December, the eve of my fortieth birthday. Buddy, my husband of then twenty years, was drifting off to sleep. While adjusting the pillows and cozying down for a restful night, my right hand meandered toward my left breast. Something wasn't right. I sat straight up. My right hand coursed the outward side of the left breast a second time. Then again and again. There was something there, a lump that was about to change the course of my life forever.

I am getting ahead of myself. There is a lot to tell and it is hard to know where to begin. It is even more difficult to know where to end. I want a perfect, "She lived happily every after" ending. Yet, if I hesitate too long, you won't get to read about the journey.

The finality of the trip is certain.
We are all terminal.
The question is when.

Journal of a Living Lady

..✍ *begins*

Journal Entry One

As Ecclesiastes says, "There is a time to live and a time to die." I have lived a good life. The hereafter should be even better.

In 1984, on the eve of my fortieth birthday, I found a lump. The next week I had a mastectomy followed by months of chemotherapy. It didn't look good. I prayed that the Lord would let me live to see our miracle son, Charlie, then age four, graduate from high school. From a medical perspective it didn't look promising, but God answered a mother's desperate prayer.

Charlie is now at Toccoa Falls College majoring in education. A fine, handsome boy he is. We also have an adopted son who is trying his wings. He crash lands now and then. I love them both and miss their daily presence at home.

After twelve years of remission, a routine doctor visit turned into my worst nightmare. The cancer had returned and spread to the lungs and lymph nodes in the middle of my chest. Metastatic breast cancer it is called.

Nothing has been the same since. Nothing ever will.

My husband, Buddy, a retired airline employee, had a fledgling computer store which he immediately shut down. We were just at a point of seeing a profit after nearly two years of struggle. One dream shot.

I had been writing a computer column for over a year for the Sentinel newspapers. It was inevitable that this had to stop also. Stress, chemotherapy and a foggy brain do not produce good copy.

My active role in the local computer club, the Civil Air Patrol and other community groups gradually ceased. Being a long-time school teacher and principal, I have always had a strong drive to teach. In spite of this illness, I have held onto teaching my Sunday School Class. This is a wonderful group of diverse, older adults. While this is my fortieth year of teaching the Bible, I know the clock is ticking toward cancer-driven retirement. Yet, I stubbornly continue to teach.

Cancer is a roller-coaster ride. Good days. Bad days. Good news. Bad news. Yesterday was "bad news" day. My oncologist told me it was now or never. I must take more chemotherapy now if I want to try to turn the tide of this cancer's aggressiveness. Otherwise, I must resign myself to palliative, symptom control.

I have vigorously resisted more chemotherapy since July. It is a "quality versus quantity" issue and I want to enjoy what time I might have left.

"Let me know when you think I am down to my last six months," I said.

Dr. Stead didn't hesitate. "Quite possibly you are there now." That was doctor number three who had indicated an expiration date before the end of year.

We are all terminal when you think about it. With cancer, there are so many issues to ponder: the physical, spiritual, emotional and financial.

I am about to give you a first-hand account of winding down. It won't be grossly morbid, I promise. My funny bone still works.

Besides, I intend to live forever. So far, so good.

Journal Entry Two

I am not a skinny model from New York. Even if I were, I wouldn't choose to be bald. Losing my hair from chemotherapy was traumatic for me. The doctor forewarned me that I'd lose it all in about two weeks. After ten days, I began to think I'd be one of the rare, but fortunate ones who didn't. Then it started. A hair here and a hair there. Then the comb brought fistfuls at a time. To keep from looking like a shedding porcupine, I had it all shaved off.

In the next two months I bought enough hats, wigs and turbans to start my own millenary shop. I didn't like any of them. They weren't the real me.

The first time I ventured to the local grocery store without any head gear, I quickly scouted the aisles. I saw nobody I knew. I was safe that day. But not always.

A bald-headed woman may as well have "cancer" or "circus lady" tattooed on her forehead. Often rude people stared. If my baldness was permitting these jerks to read my mind, they certainly weren't receiving good thoughts.

Eventually my lack of hair ceased to matter. I went everywhere, even to church, without a hat. I sat on the back row envying everybody else's hair.

Maybe it sounds trivial, but I want to have hair when I am buried, my own hair. I have never cared for anything artificial, not mock mayonnaise, not fake flowers, and especially not synthetic hair.

When I was in my twenties, I taught first grade in a little Mississippi school. A child brought *The Velveteen Rabbit* for story time. I've read it many times since.

As the story unfolds, a poignant conversation takes place in the nursery of a young boy. A well-worn rocking horse is asked by the freshly stuffed bunny rabbit, "What does it mean to be real?"

The answer given by Skin Horse gently explains one of the most fundamental truths in the universe. The bumps of life may hurt and misshapen us in the process. Yet, when the outward appearance begins to lose any semblance of beauty, our real self is revealed.

In time, the bunny rabbit became faded and worn too. The growing boy never noticed . The rabbit was his fuzzy friend, his confident, his constant companion. Then the boy got sick with scarlet fever and the contaminated rabbit was discarded. The velveteen rabbit was rescued and revived by a magical fairy. In the end, the shaggy rabbit was whole again.

Happy endings in fairy tales evoke a good feeling. Hopefulness is a buoy in real life also.

True, I have cancer. I may remain bald if I continue chemotherapy. But, it's okay, . . . really.

As the Skin Horse said, "When you are real, you can't be ugly, except to people who don't understand."

Journal Entry Three

I don't like closed places. The fancy term for it is claustrophobia. You will seldom, if ever, see me far inside a row of seats or hiding in a refrigerator.

Recently this became an issue when my doctor sent me for a MRI. Technically this is a state-of-the-art x-ray machine that gives 3-D images of body parts. Untechnically, it is more like an extra-long casket for a basketball player.

This was an older MRI machine that travels in a huge van from hospital to hospital in rural areas. The newer MRI's are more open .

After putting on a short gown that barely covered my equilateral humps, I had to lie on a narrow tray facing a dark tunnel.

"How long will I be in there?" I asked.

"About two hours in all."

"Can you get me out quickly if I call?"

"Yes," the operator said. "There's a microphone inside."

Before disappearing behind a partition, the man pushed a button that drew me slowly inside the cylinder. It was stuffy and uncomfortably snug. My shoulders involuntarily curved upward. Less than six inches distanced my nose from the ceiling. My arms were forced rigidly straight.

"Bring me out," I called loudly as my heart raced and my breathing quickened.

In seconds the table moved to the open air. "I'm sorry, but I don't know if I can do this," I said apologetically.

In the recesses of my mind was the image of an Emory University student who was buried alive in a box with a little light and a plastic air hose.

The bad guy wanted a ransom and she was underground for days. Even though the girl was eventually rescued, for weeks I had dreams about being buried alive. I never thought of it much again until this day I was in that tube.

Eventually I agreed to try again. It was a mind game. I closed my eyes and momentarily pretended I was on the beach. The MRI made a startling jack-hammer noise that jolted me to reality. I called again to come out.

On the third try I quoted everything I had ever memorized. It was amazing how lines from literature as well as passages from the Bible came to my memory.

On the fourth try, I was determined to stay. The images my doctor needed to access the spread of the cancer were completed. As I opened the door to the bright sunshine, I felt like a released prisoner.

Let it be known that when the men in the dark suits shut the top of my coffin, they had better be sure I am really dead ... I mean *dead* dead. Otherwise, Superwoman is going to raise the roof.

Journal Entry Four

As you read this, I should be kicking up sand in Florida. I may have cancer, but it doesn't have me ...not yet anyway.

While I still have enough energy to travel, I want to sit on the beach one more time. I want to watch the gorgeous sun settle somewhere in the western hemisphere and listen to the waves hitting the shore in that unrelenting rhythm.

There is something about the ocean that is absolute and calming. It is a reminder of a force we can't fathom or explain. While sitting alone, facing the endless horizon, my thoughts often turn to the serious or philosophical. Terminal illness has a way of making you face the tough issues like life and death.

When my father was dying with stomach cancer in 1982, he commented that it seemed he had only just begun his life and now it was virtually over. He was 62. Now I am in his place and I am much younger. I understand now more than ever what he meant.

Seems like just yesterday I was in grammar school sweating out my turn in the spelling bee. Where did the years go between the high school football games and the pacing off of my burial spot?

Makes me think of that scripture, "... *For what is your life? It is even a vapour, that appeareth for a little time, and then vanisheth away.*"

Will the world know that I have been here or care? I hope so. To have lived a life in vain would be a waste of God's energy.

I would like more time to leave a legacy. As the waves splash upon the shore, I am reminded that I have already had a quota of years to do just that. Life goes on and right now, somewhere, a baby is being born.

My opportunity to make a difference may soon be past. Somebody else will have a chance. Do I have any parting words for the babes of this world?

You bet.

Make every moment count. Discover the meaning of life. Give more than you take.

And, finally, take time to sit on the beach, wiggle your toes in the sand, and watch the sun set.

Journal Entry Five

Looking back through an old album, I came across my first-grade report card. The teacher commented on the back that I was a "beautiful reader." But on the inside right was a bold check mark in the behavior column. Prophetic in a way. "Claims more than her share of attention."

Here I am battling terminal cancer and writing about it. Even have a web page on the Internet. Who in their right mind would vent to the world what it is like to face death head-on? *Me.* I can't go quietly into the night. It's not my nature.

People can read about cancer. Quote statistics. Walk in the marathons. But until they have been down the cancer road, they can't fully comprehend the journey.

This past year I've lost several friends to this dread disease. James died of lung cancer. Cindee and Bob died of breast cancer. (Yes, men do get breast cancer). June and Kevon died of bone cancer. Several more of my friends, Gary, Sue, Carol, Judy, Debby, and Ray are presently fighting the big "C." The great news is that most are doing well.

I am thankful for the good months I have had. The breast cancer is on the move. We know the lungs and lymph nodes are involved and probably the spine. I've lost weight and have enough pain to warrant twenty-four hour morphine. Oxygen and home respiratory treatments have been prescribed to help breathing.

Not long ago I had a frank discussion with one of my doctors. "I am seriously considering stopping all treatment now."

He patted me on the back and told me to follow my gut feeling.I breathed a sigh of relief. This atypical physician, a primary care doctor, recognized that for some of us, the quality of remaining life is more important than quantity.

"O.K.," I said. "No more treatment." It was a personal decision not to be taken as advice for anybody else. I still want to keep my options open. Know that this decision is written in *ink*, not blood or stone. Yet, for now it is the right decision for me.

Chemotherapy makes me feel like a toxic waste dump. I have been filleted in surgery and zapped with radar guns.

Poison, slash, burn. Guess my first-grade teacher had it right. I have been pretty desperate for attention.

Journal Entry Six

What a difference two weeks make. Instead of watching the hypnotic waves of the ocean, today I am sitting in the middle of my hospital bed. No beautiful sunrises or sunsets here. Just a sterile room and a dim night light.

My right hand is laboriously trying to find the appropriate keys on the laptop computer. My left hand wants to join in, but my defiant fingers refuse to uncurl. The doctors aren't sure whether this is a mini-stroke or a further complication of the cancer going bodily north this time.

Doctor Rob and my husband, Buddy, have started the hospice process. Later I will share more details about this organization for the terminally ill. Buddy understands now that he can't carry this load alone. He insists that he doesn't want me in an institution…that he wants me constantly near-by and that that he married me "until death do us part." While he will continue to be my primary caregiver, hospice will provide him with additional support personnel.

Quite often people ask Buddy about visiting in our home. He loves company and so do I most of the time. However, my Buddy has this strange need to take every guest on a walking tour of our humble abode.

Take my word for it. Martha Stewart and her finery winery dinery would be out of place in our home. However, should she show up at our door, Buddy would take great delight in giving her the grand tour. This generally includes removing the porcelain toilet cover to demonstrate how well the ball floats. Never mind that my unmentionables are drying on the shower bar.

Understand that I didn't grow up in high society, but I do have a little pride. No matter how desperately ill I am, if I know you are coming, I will attempt to clean house. It is an unwritten "woman" thing.

Oppie, our Chihuahua, and Rocky, our parrot, contribute to our daily household debris. But it is really those night creatures that keep our house untidy. I read about them in Grime's Book of Fairies.

They do their dirty deeds when everybody else is asleep. Ms. Grime Fairy uses a waxy wand to leave marks in the bath tubs and toilets. Her sister, Ms. Dust Fairy, goes into each room depositing powdery droppings on all tables, shelves and what-knots. If you aren't seeing evidences of the Grime Fairies at your house, then you have a maid or a lot more energy than I have.

You won't see our house on the Christmas Tour of Homes. You won't be able to eat off our floors. You may have to help yourself to the refrigerator and I may take a nap if you stay long. But *real* friends are welcome anytime.

Journal Entry Seven

A paradox is a term that is seemingly absurd or contradictory, but is really founded on truth. For example, time is a great teacher, but it has a way of killing all of its students.

An oxymoron is a combination of contradictory or incongruous words like small crowd, jumbo shrimp, civil war, and serious fun.

While some might argue that I am dying with cancer, the truth of the matter is that I am *living* with it. Even though I am a realist and understand the grim statistics for advanced metastatic cancer, I still have hope. I believe in miracles. Yet, it is not God's will for everyone to live forever in these mortal and imperfect bodies.

A few days ago I agreed to be enrolled in a hospice program. Hospice is reserved for people who are believed to be in their last six months of life as determined by a physician.

When Dr. Rob first suggested hospice, I told him I had rather wait until I was closer to the end of that hypothetical six-month period. My idea of a hospice patient was one who was totally bed-ridden, foggy-minded and in need of hourly monitoring.

Hospice seems to be a good choice. In a recent survey, nine out of ten people said they would prefer to die at home and not in sterile, impersonal surroundings hooked up by tubes to machines. The founder of the modern hospice movement summed up its philosophy succinctly, "You matter to the last moment of your life, and we will do all we can, not only to help you die peacefully, but to live until you die."

Oncologists are now recommending that a patient enter a hospice program earlier in a life-limiting illness rather than later. One reason is that there is so much preliminary paperwork. Much of it involves insurance, Medicare, and legal matters. There are endless questions which I would prefer to answer now while I am nearly sane.

Buddy should not have to make weighty decisions while under emotional duress like who he should marry next. I am afraid that if he were hungry enough, he would probably choose the first widow who brought him a big bowl of banana pudding.

A few months ago a good friend, a widow, called to tell me she wanted to give me a farewell party. She excitedly rattled on and on about her plans which included inviting innumerable friends and relatives.

While she had the best of intentions, I tactfully declined. What could possibly be said after "Good-bye, nice knowing you." Maybe the butler would contribute something memorable like, "Here, have another piece of chopped liver for us to remember Nancy."

And what would everybody sing? The Hallelujah Chorus? I know what I would be saying. "Ashes to ashes, dust to dust. Get off my oxygen line or I'm going to bust."

This party thing was a nice gesture on my friend's part, but for now I have a more pressing priority: Breathe in, breathe out!

Journal Entry Eight

The Statue of Liberty is the only woman in the U.S. who is positive she will never get breast cancer. Approximately 181,000 people are diagnosed annually with breast cancer and 44,000 die from it.

These are the figures just for breast cancer. Think of all the other forms of cancer and we are talking some mind-numbing numerics. I've never been a mathematical wizard. Long-haired professors of the 1960's left me mathematically challenged with their circular eyeglasses, square pies and rhythm methods for logs.

Yet, I've served my academic time with cardinal numbers, cube roots, minuends, Roman numerals, and trigonometric functions. Even crunched a few bits and bytes.

But if you want to discuss absolutes and infinity, come on over. I know the mathematician of all mathematicians. In Psalms, it is written, "*He apointeth the number of the stars; he calleth them all by their names.*" I think that if God knows the name of each and every star, I can rest in peace knowing he knows my name and yours too. If we are honest, most of us like to be called by our names.

One of my physicians takes the time to call me on the phone and gives me lab reports in person. He asks me how I'm doing and he's not just wanting to pass time. He wants to know how I *really* am. There is compassion there which I greatly appreciate.

What I don't like is to call a doctor's office and get some receptionist who has probably never even driven past a medical school. Yet, she tries to diagnose the intricacies of metastatic cancer on the telephone.

"And just where is your pain?"

She wouldn't want me to really answer that. Finally, after twenty questions, we get to the point that she thinks my problem might need to be discussed with the doctor. She leaves me waiting while she checks her schedule book.

"O. K., Mrs. Kelly. The first appointment we have is three weeks from today at 4:45 p.m. Is that O.K.?"

"No," I answer politely, thinking that I'll either be dead or well in that length of time.

"Is there anyone else there I can talk to?" I ask, hoping for her supervisor.

"Sorry." the receptionist replies. "There's nobody here with higher authority."

Journal Entry Nine

Alternative isn't an immoral word though it does seem to have some sinister connotation. You don't usually find the scholarly, well-behaved child in an alternative school. The alternative is generally not as good as our first choice. And then there is alternative medicine. I am still not sure what "established" medical practice means either. Everyday brings conflicting advice.

It is a bit unnerving to me that doctors call what they do *practice*. The last time I lay waiting my turn in the surgical suite swigging Valium, I cupped my ear to hear the muffled voices in the inner sanctum. I am almost sure I overhead someone say, "Hey, there's big money in kidneys these days and this gal has two of them."

Ever since it has become common knowledge that I have serious cancer, I have had some sincere people and some sincerely strange people offer me alternatives to traditional medicine.

I honestly believe there is good in both traditional and alternative medicine, so don't shoot the messenger here. I may not have much time left as it is.

Having cancer can cause desperate irrationality. I have tried it all, right down to the worming medicine.

First there was this lady with the frantic voice who called one morning. "Are you the lady with cancer?"

"One of them," I answered cautiously.

"Can I come to your house. I won't take much time, I promise. You just must know about the secret tea that has cured 1,000's of cancer patients."

She came. She stayed. And I paid. The special tea had to be precisely made and then be strained. After a few hours, it had to be strained again. I have often wished that Lucille Ball could have lived long enough to have filmed this ridiculous ritual. It would have been her finest segment ever.

In the past several months, I have tried every promising pill, liquid, powder or grassy herb that could, should or would cure cancer. The I hit my lowest low and did what I vowed I would never do. Remember that desperate people do desperate things.

The easy part was brewing the strongest coffee that Columbia can legally ship. It had to be thoroughly chilled before using.

I am a proper lady and don't know how to politely explain the procedure. Be glad I'm not a good artist either. Just think of a five-letter word that starts and ends with vowels. (Hint: e & a)

Behind the privacy of a four-way locked bathroom door, I positioned the paraphernalia needed to accomplish the task. Would this hundred-proof coffee cleaner do as promised … cure my cancer?

I took a deep breath and courageously released the valve. Moments later I wished Lucille Ball *was* there in my place.

In hind-sight, I wouldn't do it again. Yes, I lived for another day. And another. But I am not proud of it. In doing so, I have become the Queen of Gullibility.

Who writes these self-help books anyway?

Journal Entry Ten

The year of 1949 must have been a bumper year for weddings. It is unbelievable how many of our friends are celebrating their 50th anniversary this year. It is a good thing that giving gifts for reaching the half century mark in marriage is no longer socially apropos. The only gold I have is in my teeth.

Last week Buddy and I celebrated our 34th wedding anniversary. We met in a Baptist church in Memphis in the early sixties. Several months later we married. In all these years, we have never seriously considered divorce, just murder.

The success of our marriage is largely due to Buddy's patient temperament. If we were four-legged, I'd be a spirited Tennessee Walking horse and he'd be a lovable, loyal Mississippi mule. Though our personalities are different, our values are much the same. He can practically read my mind and I quite often finish his sentences. Though we are two, we are one.

I cannot picture life without Buddy. He can't fathom life without me. This cancer thing is hard to deal with emotionally for both of us. Sometimes I glance at a family picture and experience an unexpected rush of tears. Buddy takes long walks and angrily kicks loose rocks along the way. After fostering a dozen kids, adopting one, and then finally getting our own son off to college, we looked forward to a peaceful retirement. This recurrence of cancer was a most *un*welcome shock.

Terminal disease has a way of awakening a marriage even if it was already good. Spontaneous hugs come at odd times in odd places. Late at night, I often leave my hospital bed in the spare room and climb into bed with Buddy. Only then can either of us sleep soundly. We belong together.

Buddy and I had the word "Mizpah" put on our wedding cake. It was also engraved in our wedding bands. It will be on the ribbon that drapes my coffin. Mizpah is a Hebrew word taken from Genesis which means, "*The Lord watch between me and thee when we are absent one from another.*"

Cancer cannot cripple our love or change eternity. Buddy and I will remain together until death do us part. Then, after a little while, we will be together again. So help me, God.

Journal Entry Eleven

*I*t is almost midnight and the hospital hallways are eerily quiet. I've been here nearly two weeks now, but will be checking out in the morning after my last radiation treatment.

What began as a scheduled doctor visit turned into a prolonged nightmare. Sicker than sick, I was immediately escorted to the hospital. The staff by-passed the normal admission procedures. Only one hitch: the semi-private room.

Two of us were coming in about the same time. Both emergency admits. Both with the same first name. *One* was crazy.

"What are you in for?" I asked, trying to make conversation.

"Dope, I guess. Diabetes too," she said. Her life story poured out, mingled with graphic expletives. Before long, I realized I should not have worn my black skirt with the white turtle top. Evidently Crazy Jane mistook me for a nun.

"Don't tell any of these nurses that I am a doper. You promise?"

"Scout's honor," I said, knowing full well I wasn't going to be staying the night with this wild woman. Crazy Jane pulled the sheet used for a room divider back and forth continuously as she told bits and pieces about her life.

"Been doping for a long time," she confessed. "They're looking for me, you know. Don't tell them, sister."

"Tell them what?" I asked.

"Where I've been and where I am going."

I smiled in reply.

My bed was closest to the door. When the floor nurse came in, I grabbed the bottom pocket of her smock.

"Will you please get me out of here," I whispered. This woman is not in her right mind."

The hefty nurse gave me a rather self-righteous look over her half-moon glasses. "Not a private room in the whole hospital, my dear."

Soon two young nurse wantabees came in asking their long list of rapid-fire questions:

"Do you smoke?"

"No," I tersely replied, irritated that there wasn't a private room available. "A person with cancer would be crazy to smoke."

Crazy Jane broke in, "Well, I smoke." she laughed. "Why quit now?"

Both of us were asked if we abused alcohol. Crazy Jane admitted to being a heavy drinker. I disavowed any association with wine or liquor of any sorts.

When asked if either of us used illegal drugs, I again said, no. Crazy Jane lied. I was loyal to my word. I didn't rat on her.

Then came the most asinine question of all. "How many times have you been to the bathroom today?"

Crazy Jane responded innocently, "Number one or number two?"

Now I giggled. The aide got no answer from me on that one. I didn't know how many times I had gone to the bathroom. I don't tally such things Besides, I was too sick to care.

Eventually Crazy Jane became more hyperactive. She made rude comments to passer-bys in the hallway. The nurse who had been so snooty before came back and whispered that they had found a place for me. "It isn't exactly a room," she murmured, glancing toward the other side of the sheet.

"Does it have a bed?" I asked.

"Yes, if an examining bed counts."

"Does it have a toilet?"

"Yes, but it does not have a shower."

"I'll take it. I'll take it," I said, trying to muffle my excitement.

Just then a telephone call came in from Crazy Jane's ex-husband. Apparently he had gotten out of jail in Texas and was on the way to see her.

I hastily packed up my few things. As I headed toward the door, Crazy Jane put the phone receiver on the bed and ran to give me a big hug, complete with a wet kiss on the cheek.

"Thanks for moving out. My ex and I have so much catching up to do after three years." She gave me a wink as she hurried back to the phone.

"See you in church next week," I said jokingly.

Crazy Jane replied. "Just might see me there, sister. You just might."

Journal

of a

Living Lady

continues

Journal Entry Twelve

*I*f someone told you that they had found a fork in the road, what would you think? That some careless person had lost an eating utensil or that some philosopher had come to choices in his path? I've discovered lately that there are some practical and creative uses for something as simple and mundane as a fork.

This story isn't folklore. Like me, there was a lady diagnosed with a terminal illness. I'll call her Lydia. She had been given three months to live. Lydia was getting things in order as most of us do when we enter the "count-down" to the end of life. She asked her pastor to come to her home to discuss final wishes.

Lydia told the pastor which songs she wanted sung at her funeral service. She showed him the scriptures that she desired to be read. Lydia also requested that she be buried with her favorite Bible. The pastor wrote all her requests in his little black note-book.

"There's one more thing," she added excitedly. "I want to be buried with a fork in my right hand."

The puzzled pastor raised his heavy eyebrows. Lydia noted his surprise. "Well, let me explain it, pastor. In all my years of attending church meetings, socials, fund-raisers and potluck dinners, I always remember that when the dishes of the main course were being cleared, someone would inevitably lean over and say, 'Keep your fork.'

"Keeping the fork was my favorite part because I knew something better was coming like velvety chocolate cake or deep-dish apple pie with ice cream. It was always something good and worth waiting for. So, I just want people to see me there in that casket with a fork in my hand. I want them to wonder what the fork is for. Then I want you to tell them: 'Keep your fork. The best is yet to come!' "

The pastor's eyes welled up with tears of joy as he hugged the woman good-bye. He knew this could be last time he might see her before her death. He also knew that the woman had a clearer view of heaven than most in his congregation. She knew that something better was coming.

At the funeral, people walked by Lydia's casket. She wore a beautiful pink gown. Her heavily-marked Bible laid beside her. A silver fork was tightly gripped in her right hand.

Over and over, the pastor heard the question, "What's with the fork?" He smiled and replied that he would explain later. During the service, the pastor told about the fork and what it symbolized to Lydia. She knew in her heart that the best is yet to come.

Journal Entry Thirteen

*O*bviously I am still living or you'd be reading my obituary. I don't like funerals, but obituaries fascinate me. Not that I'm glad somebody died, of course. I am just curious. Who died? What caused their death? How old were they? What did they accomplish in life?

Mother Teresa was 87 when she died. Frank Sinatra was 82. Methuselah lived 900 years.

Yogi Berra had some advice about funerals. He said to always go to other people's funerals. Otherwise, they won't come to yours.

A friend told me about a grave stone she read that said,

"Pause, stranger, when you pass me by,
As you are now, so once was I.
As I am now, so will you be;
So prepare for death and follow me."

A tourist put this at the bottom of the inscription,

"To follow you I am not content
Until I know which way you went."

Have you ever wondered what would be written on your headstone? I've thought about it lately. My philosophical side would want, "*There are no luggage racks on a hearse*." My educational inclination would favor "*A teacher to the last.*" My spiritual leaning would persuade me to choose, *"Home at last."* What is etched in stone isn't really that important. In actuality, we are writing our epitaphs everyday we live.

Buddy and I have had a good marriage. If he were to go

before me, I'd really miss him and all those little things he does for me that I tend to take for granted. He tells me that he will greatly miss me. I hope so or I would have failed miserably in matrimony.

Words to a song from the Great Gatsby fills my mind:

"What'll I do when you are far away and I
am blue, what'll I do?
What'll I do with just a photograph to tell
my troubles to.
What'll I do with only dreams of you that
won't come true, What'll I do?"

In time, Buddy will be okay after I'm gone. He knows death is part of living and that I've had my bags packed for this journey for a long time. So has he. Because of our spiritual faith, we take comfort in knowing that our separation will only be temporary. In the meanwhile, I'll keep fighting this cancer and he'll keep holding my hand.

Recently I saw a sign in a plant nursery that caught my attention. It said, "*Our plants are guaranteed to live or die trying.*" Yet, I have a platitude that beats it: "*I am going to live forever. Not even dying can stop me.*"

None of us can live this life but once, but if we do it right, once is enough. Then comes life's graduation.

Journal Entry Fourteen

Though I also have metastatic breast cancer, this is not my story. I do know that it is true account. Oft repeated, it has to be shared.

"My grandparents were married for over half a century and played their own special game from the time they had met each other. The goal of their game was to write the word "shmily" in a surprise place for the other to find. They took turns leaving "shmily" around the house. As soon as one of them discovered it, it was their turn to hide it once more.

They dragged "shmily" with their fingers through the sugar and flour containers, to await whoever was preparing the next meal. They smeared it in the dew on the windows overlooking the patio, where my grandma always fed us warm, homemade pudding with blue food coloring.

"Shmily" was written in the steam left on the mirror after a hot shower, where it would reappear bath after bath. At one point, my grandmother even unrolled an entire roll of toilet paper, to leave "shmily" on the very last sheet. There was no end to the places "shmily" would pop up. Little notes with "shmily" scribbled hurriedly were found on dashboards and car seats or taped to steering wheels. The notes were stuffed inside shoes and left under pillows. "Shmily" was written in the dust upon the mantel and traced in the ashes of the fireplace.

This mysterious word was as much a part of my grandparents' house as the furniture. It took me a long time before I was able to fully appreciate my grandparents' game. Skepticism had kept me from believing in true love - one that is pure and enduring. However, I never doubted my grandparents' relationship. They had love down pat. It was more than their flirtatious little games; it was a way of life Their relationship was based on devotion and passionate affection: quick kisses as they bumped into each other in their tiny kitchen, finishing each other's sentences, sharing the daily crossword puzzle and word jumble.

My grandma whispered to me about how cute my grandpa was, how handsome he had grown to be. She claimed that she really knew "how to pick 'em." Before every meal, they bowed their heads and gave thanks, marveling at their blessings: a wonderful family, good fortune, and each other.

However, there was dark cloud in my grandparents' lives: my grandmother had breast cancer. The disease had first appeared ten years earlier. As always, Grandpa was with her every step of the way. He comforted her in their yellow room, painted that way so she could always be surrounded by sunshine, even when she was too sick to go outside.

Now the cancer was again attacking her body. With the help of a cane and my grandfather's steady hand, they went to church every Sunday morning. My grandmother grew steadily weaker until, finally, she could not leave the house anymore. For a while, Grandpa would go to church alone, praying to God watch over his wife.

Then one day, what we all dreaded finally happened. Grandma was gone. "Shmily" was scrawled in yellow on the pink ribbons of my grandmother's funeral bouquet. As the crowd thinned and the last mourners turned to leave, my aunts, uncles, cousins and other family members came forward and gathered around Grandma one last time.

Grandpa stepped up to my grandmother's casket. Taking a shaky breath, he began to sing to her. Through his tears and grief, the song came, a deep and throaty lullaby. Shaking with my own sorrow, I will never forget that moment. I knew that, although I couldn't begin to fathom the depth of their love, I had been privileged to witness its unmatched beauty."

S-H-M-I-L-Y: See How Much I Love you.

Journal Entry Fifteen

Everyone wants to know about *the* reunion. It has taken me a couple of weeks to come down from the high of visiting around the clock for two days with over thirty relatives from seven states. Some of these kinfolk I hadn't seen since early childhood. Funny how you remember people as you last saw them. Curly-headed Jackie was now bald John. Change is inevitable, except from vending machines.

The recently founded Making Memories Organization granted me their first wish as a terminal breast cancer patient. I mentioned to a friend on the Internet weeks ago that if I could have a last wish, it would be for a reunion with my extended family *before* the funeral, not afterwards. That way I could get in on the party. Not long after, I received a wonderful phone call from the Executive Director, Fran Hansen, saying the organization wanted to grant my wish.

Our phone bill was over $150 last month, but it was worth every penny as I contacted relatives to see if they could come. Not only did they desire to come, they wanted to bring all the nieces, nephews and cousins. We even had a great, great nephew present at the reunion as well as three newborns.

While the Making Memories organization originally offered to pay for a cottage and couple of rooms, the number of relatives wanting to come kept expanding. I have never been good at saying no. I soon began making diagrams of who could sleep back to back without fighting. The overflow had to sleep at our home a couple of miles away, but it worked out fine.

A limousine company donated one of those stretch black cars that the rich and famous ride in. It was my first and probably last limo ride unless you call a hearse a limousine. Maybe it is the family who rides in the hearse. I don't know what they call the corpse car. I eschew obfuscation.

Just before approaching the entrance of the Brasstown Valley Resort, a man jumped out of a television truck. He opened the limousine door and ran a microphone cord down my back. From then on everything I said was on tape. I was hoping to get a chance to give a "heads up" to all the relatives waiting for me at the resort portal. I did not want them to say or do anything outrageous on national television as in the Jerry Springer style. My maiden name is "White," but we aren't white trash. Yet, you know the old saying, "Familiarity breeds attempt."

I was greeted at the Brasstown entrance with a dozen red roses and hugs from my sons, three brothers and my only sister, Sunnie Anne. In the foreground were scores of relatives and friends waving and crying tears of joys. The big network cameras were there and lots of national and local reporters. It is said that everybody gets five minutes of fame in life. I got about two hours.

All the interview questions were reasonable except for the first two asked of my sister: "Would you call this a salvage operation?" and "Is this event like the Phoenix rising from the ashes?" I sure was glad Sunnie Anne got those questions and not me. The whole event seemed like something from a fairy tale. Davis Palmour presented me with a "Nancy Kelly Day" plaque from the city of Young Harris and read the resolution like a courtly prince. Buddy assisted me to a waiting wheelchair and Kay Raymond from the Chamber of Commerce and Dale Rice from the resort escorted the family to a back room for further surprises.

With all the spotlights on me, someone turned on a long audio tape that sounded just like my friend, Patsy Rahn, whom I had previously asked to sing at my funeral. Even Buddy leaned over and asked if that was Patsy. I nodded that I thought so. It certainly sounded like her.

With the cameras coming in for a close-up, Kay asked me to tell everybody the background of the lyrics just played. I must have looked like a dumb-founded plucked chicken. What words? I hadn't paid attention to the lyrics, partly because I was in still in shock and partly because I was concentrating on identifying the singer.

Thankfully, my sister, who was standing behind me, came to my rescue. She leaned over my shoulder and whispered, "Knowing Nancy." It immediately rung my ringer and kept me from babbling like Goofus.

During the wee hours of the reunion morning, volunteer professionals in Dallas had set a stranger's poem to music. The tape had arrived at the Brasstown Resort at 3:00 a.m. by Federal Express.

Several days earlier, Bob Cleveland from Alabama, had read my newspaper columns and wrote a beautiful poem using the initials of my whole name as an acronym. When I received it in the mail, I was so impressed with his thoughtfulness that I forwarded a copy of "Knowing Nancy" via e-mail to Sunnie Anne. She recognized the lyrics in the song.

Believe me, I am not a celebrity or heroine. Knowing me and one dollar will get you a cup of coffee in most any restaurant. I can't help but wonder how I was chosen for such a special day. After all, my only claim to fame is having metastatic breast cancer. There are *lots* of ladies, and men too, who have breast cancer. I didn't deserve all this attention.

My only hope is that when this organization is nationally spotlighted, generous people will contribute to this worthy cause. The reunion helped me forget about breast cancer for a couple of days and gave me some truly cherished memories.

Good things still happen to common people.

Journal of a Living Lady

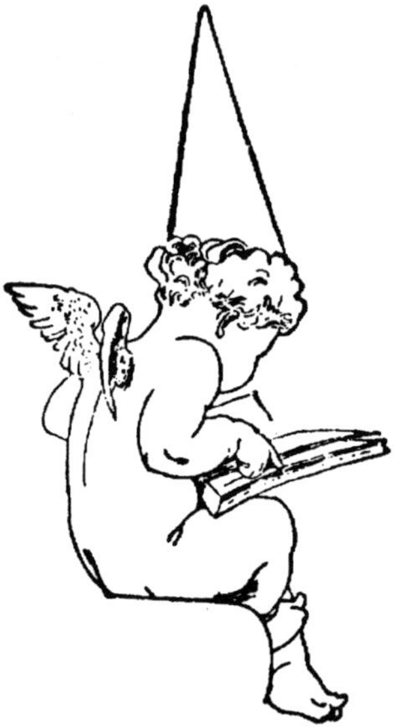

continues

Journal Entry Sixteen

How do you write a newspaper column? Word by word. Line by line. Literally. Not always though is it *this* difficult.

Recently I returned home from another week in the hospital. I can barely stay vertical for more than ten minutes at a time.

The increased bone pain required more radiation. Radiation zaps energy. There is hardly an ounce of vitality in my body. An internal port was surgically implanted in my chest for chemotherapy. Add soreness to no energy. Picking up a glass of tea requires pitiful effort.

Several months ago I decided to forgo more treatment. Yet, pain is a tremendous mind-changer. To silence the pain of cancer, we patients give in and consequently give up more cognitive skills than we would like. Previously I backed off most pain medications thinking I was over the hump. Then the truly difficult pain hit. It took high doses of meds in the hospital to get back to tolerable levels of pain.

Three weeks ago I was laughing and hugging relatives at a happy family reunion. Those two days I didn't feel very sick at all. I certainly felt no pain.

Today I look like an emaciated prisoner of war. Thankfully I am stronger than yesterday. I will come out of this again. I am still not ready to go gently into the night. As long as I have breath, I have purpose. I keep repeating that mantra as I drift off to sleep. A couple of times I have wondered if I would awaken again, but I did, of course. Rousing to a new day is my confirmation that God intends for me to keep living. He is in charge of my medical situation. I just have to stay the course and trust His purpose in all of this. There is a reason behind the circumstances in our lives. Nothing happens to God's children by accident.

I am in a refining process. No doubt I am a somewhat better person because of this disease. Refining gold is not an easy process. Pound. Mix. Scrub. Roll. Melt. Treat with acid. It is all necessary for the end result.

Most of us know the story of Job. God allowed Satan to do as he wished with him except take his life. In spite of all the calamities that came his way, Job maintained his integrity. He never vented his anger toward God. "*Through all this Job did not sin by charging God with any wrongdoing.*" (Job 1:22)

God is our Maker. His wisdom is far beyond our finite minds. While we cannot see the whole picture, He can. If I am to be of any use in his masterful plan, then I understand his need to refine me.

Michelangelo, a renowned sculptor of days long ago, loved to work with marble. An eight foot statute of David is said to have been his favorite sculpture. I can vouch for its magnificence. I have seen and touched the great work myself.

While Michelangelo was chiseling on this massive project, much of the pristine white marble fell away. The people who sweated to bring the marble to the work site complained loudly. To them it was an unconscionable waste.

Michelangelo could see what other could not. He calmly responded to the unjust criticism: "*As the chips fall away, the image emerges.*"

Journal Entry Seventeen

My last column found me gently knocking on death's door. Fortunately, or maybe unfortunately, the hinges stubbornly refused to budge. As my strength returns, I see no entourage of angels. Certainly no grim reaper. Just laundry and dirty dishes.

Dr. Stead, my oncologist, just called to remind me I need chemotherapy to help contain the bone metastasis. She asked *when* I was coming in, not *if*. I told her I was still trying to psyche myself up for it. I think she knew I wouldn't call her first.

Dr. Nancy White Stead is a brilliant, petite, lively, young doctor who is married to a surgeon. You would never suspect that she is a physician to see her in street clothes away from a medical setting. Though quite professional, she has an innocent, bubbly personality with a unique girlish voice.

My first impression of her two years ago was that she would be a good model for a Barbie doctor set. After she gave me my initial new patient physical, I came away confident that I was in very competent hands. She found every crease, crack, spot and orifice I have. If Dr. Stead needed a second job, she would make a great strip search officer for illicit drugs.

After carefully answering all my questions regarding the side effects of Aredia, Dr. Stead convinced me to come in Monday. Buddy is going to take our light-weight recliner because the drip takes four hours. At least this particular chemotherapy won't cause me lose my hair. It's supposed to make me feel like I have the flu for a few days. Then in a month I get to do it all over again.

Guess I have learned to never say never. Until the pain became intolerable, my plan was to ride this paling horse to the end of the trail. There would be no further surgery, radiation or chemotherapy. I reneged.

Last month I agreed to more surgery to replace my

porta-cath. A second round of radiation zapped the spine. Now comes more of the dreaded chemotherapy.

We have a creek that runs through our property. On Monday morning I will go outside and look for a frog in the creek. Somebody told me that if you eat a live frog in the morning, nothing worse will happen to either of you the rest of the day.

Journal Entry Eighteen

My mind is always making contracts my body can't keep. I want to do so many things and actually plan to do them. Then reality sets in. Two or three hours at a time are about all I can handle without a good nap. There are lots of places where I can't conveniently nap like when driving the car, sitting at the dinner table with friends or while shopping for groceries. Probably I could stretch out in the meat counter, but a little ole lady might have trouble rolling me over to get to the ground beef.

It's hard to distinguish what is related to the cancer and what is simply related to older age. Some days it seems that everything hurts and what doesn't hurt doesn't work well. I am certainly better than I was a month ago, but not nearly where I want to be. Most times I feel like the "morning after" even though I haven't been anywhere or done anything.

Both my maternal grandmother and my mother used to say on days they didn't feel well, "I just have to make myself do." That is what I find myself doing…making myself do, go, read and even write.

It would be easy to stay in bed. Someone with terminal cancer certainly has reason enough to lay low and withdraw from life. It is a battle some mornings to put two feet on the floor. I know the day may come when I can't *will* myself to keep going. But I'm not there yet.

The only difference I see between a rut and a grave is the depth. When you are in a hole, you don't just sit. With every ounce of strength you have left, you struggle to hoist yourself from the pit.

We can't forget in the dark what we've learned in the light. Another day means another opportunity to make a difference in the life of somebody else. We shouldn't go through life with a catchers mitt on both hands. We need to be able to throw something back. I don't want any part of an empty life. We have meaning and purpose as long as we breathe.

Yesterday is gone. Tomorrow may never come. But we have today and that is what matters.

Someone said, "Don't sweat the petty things." We should not linger to pet the sweaty things either. We must keep on keeping on long after we can't.

I am off to the grocery store now. If I am not back in two hours, I told Buddy to look for me in the horizontal frozen food bin.

Journal Entry Nineteen

The acoustics in the doctor's waiting room were undeniably poor. Talks with the busy receptionist, interchanges between nurses, all phone calls in and out and even dialogue between waiting patients were easily heard by all.

My chemotherapy which was scheduled for a two hour intake kept me six hours. Dr. Stead and her staff grew more and more behind. Waiting forces you to observe all that is going on around you.

In the foyer was a young woman with short, unevenly cropped hair. That usually means recovery from chemotherapy. The strongest chemo takes your hair in about ten days. I have been totally hairless twice. The only good thing about being bald is that you don't have to worry about being dragged off by a caveman.

The frail girl and I mutually smiled as each of us pulled out a copy of the same thick book we had brought to read. I read about ten pages of *The Visitation* by Frank Peretti and then put it up. She was still reading late that afternoon.

The eerie quietness of the waiting room was interrupted by a weak, but antagonistic voice. It came from the lab area. "No. Don't. I don't want to. Stop." It was hard to discern whether this was a child resisting blood being drawn or someone much older. The nurse was sympathetic and condoling.

"Won't you let me try? Just one stick and it'll be all over." In a few seconds the nurse commented in a comforting voice, "Well, it's all done now. No more sticks." We all breathed a sigh of relief.

Everyone waited to see the one who dared to voice opposition to the expected needle sticks. A bent, fragile-looking elderly lady emerged clutching a small teddy bear. She was assisted by a barely younger sister and a man. The old woman staggered and almost fell. The sister and man instinctively hooked their arms inside her spindly ones to steady her. She was walking death.It took little imagination to envision her stretched out in a coffin.

A couple, probably in their late sixties, awaited their own visit with Dr. Stead. They stared intently as the threesome slowly exited the front door. Tears welled up in the eyes of the balding man who had been reading a church bulletin. He looked at his wife who responded with a tearful wince. I wondered if their visual exchange was pity for the old lady or the often thought question, "Is that what I will look like soon?" Maybe both.

This is the way you think in cancer wards and treatment centers. You look at everybody else and wonder how far along in the journey they are. You see stages you once were and stages you imagine you will see in the future. I wasn't as far along as the frail, old lady, but probably much further down the road than the young girl with the cropped hair. I left the office late in the afternoon totally drained from the chemotherapy and the real-life drama I had just witnessed.

I thought of Carl Sandburg who said, "*Life is like an onion; you peel off one layer at a time and sometimes you weep.*" Thankfully, there are other quotes that make us smile in dark times:

"*God is dead.*" ... Nietchze
"*Nietchze is dead.*" ... **God**

Journal Entry Twenty

VENI, VIDI, VISA used to be my motto: "I came, I saw, I shopped." I could never pass a yard sale or flea market without my brakes screeching to a stop. My right turns were never made with precision at such speed. I once took a mail box down in my enthusiasm.

Neither Buddy nor I enjoy shopping like we used to. Part of it is that we no longer have children in the home to surprise with little gifts or new clothes.

The second reason is that in the process of growing older, we have found that accumulating things, or *stuff* as our pastor calls it, isn't what is important in life. He who dies with the most toys nevertheless is dead.

The third reason we don't shop much anymore is because we don't have the disposable income we had in our working years. With a son in college, plus medical bills, frugality has become a necessity. It's not hard for us to meet expenses. They are everywhere.

Actually, we have all we need and don't need all we want. We may not have a Better Homes and Garden house, but it is adequate and paid for. Our clothes didn't come from Neiman Marcus, but labels never meant much to us anyway. Our vehicles are long out of warranty, but are still dependable.

Considering who you compare us with, Donald Trump or Freddie the Freeloader, we could be ranked on either end of the prosperity scale. My father used to tell us children that if we had a roof over our heads, could pay our bills on time, had food on the table and had at least a dollar left over, we were rich. According to that definition we are theoretically wealthy. Practically, we are not.

New Millenium issues don't bother us. We do not have hoards of money to withdraw from the bank. Neither are we worried about stock crashes. Our three shares of stock won't make or break us. Our treasures aren't buried in the hills near a certain old tree.

Money has its place in life. It is not the root of all evils. The *love* of it is. Financial wealth is a lousy way of keeping score. It's not what you have in life that counts; it is *who* you have in your life. There's nothing in this world worth trading for God, family or good friends.

Journal Entry Twenty-One

Funny thing about deadlines. They make a swooshing sound as they go by. It is time to write my weekly column again and my mind is blank. In journalism, they call it writer's block. Every author experiences this now and then. My remedy is to pretend that there is glue in my seat.

One thing I have learned in life is that inspiration plus motivation is 98% perspiration. Consequently, when writer's block occurs, I do not answer the phone. I do not raid the refrigerator. I do not exaggerate the call of nature. Not until I have at least one hundred words written will I reluctantly acknowledge my cat's pleading meow. The last one is the hardest. If you have ever owned a cat, or had a cat own you, you understand.

Mo Mo, our Himalayan kitten, always demands attention. Never is she as adamant though as when I am seriously writing. She knows when I have a dead-line. It doesn't matter.

Mo Mo is a self-centered schemer who must have her way. You would think a veteran school teacher and principal who has handled the most undisciplined of children could dominate a little cat.

Mo Mo jumps in my lap. I push her down. She jumps again. I push her down once more. After sever unsuccessful attempts to stay put in my lap, she waits a few seconds and defiantly jumps up there once again. This time Mo Mo has a plan. She lays on her back and looks like a dead fluffy rag. She purrs contently as her paw gently strokes my face. Who can resist such charm? I caress her long silky hair and scratch behind her ears.

All mama cats give their children the *Kitten Play Book* when they are born. It is downloaded with their milk. That is why all cats know how to play the same manipulative games with their owners. I even over-heard one mama cat teaching her kittens a bit of feline history: "*Thousands of years ago, cats were worshipped as gods. Never forget this.*"

Wonderful. Mo Mo just jumped down from my lap and has left my little office. Quality time. That was all she needed. Now I can *finally* get on with my writing.

No such luck. Here comes Mo Mo again. Now she is doing the two-step on the computer keyboard leaving traces of kitty litter between the keys. Her next trick will be to double-click my computer mouse.

When I lock her in the spare bedroom, she jumps at anything not nailed down causing enough commotion for me to come running. If I put her outside, she climbs on the window screen and becomes Mo Mo, the Ripper.

I have tried to ignore or out-stubborn this two-pound mass of purring insistence. Mo Mo always wins. She doesn't just have a plan "B" to get my attention. She has strategies all the way to "Z." Right now she is pawing the cordless phone buttons, creating zany musical tunes.

I give up. Today I will just enjoy my adorable, obnoxious cat.

Journal Entry Twenty-Two

Being two weeks past chemotherapy and feeling a little better, the inevitable happened. Ocean itch struck again. There is something about the sea that draws me to it. I can't explain it. I just have to go once in a while if for no other reason than to make sure it is still there.

Last week we took a spur of the moment trip to Myrtle Beach. Using the computer, I went on-line and checked out priceline.com. Here you can make a bid on a plane ticket or a motel room. If your bid is accepted, you are booked. No refunds. No changes in dates. You can't choose your motel, but you can request a certain star rating which protects you from the hole-in-the road types. For $38 plus tax we got a confirmation for two nights in the middle of the week.

I packed suitcases and counted out a three-day supply of pills. Buddy loaded up the car with the heavy-duty oxygen machine I sleep under at night plus lots of portable O2 bottles. We headed out at 6:00 in the morning and figured on being there around lunch time. It didn't look that far on the map. We made it to our destination as the sun was setting.

The motel was actually a condominium/resort hotel complete with kitchen and ocean-view balcony. We were too tired to do anything that night except go to bed. We were still too road weary to do much the next day. I did take a brief stroll down the windy beach and collected a few shells while Buddy snoozed.

We paid $50 plus a tip to eat in one of those all you can eat seafood restaurants. I ate about $3 worth. Just to say we did something while on vacation, Buddy checked into one of the live country shows. It didn't start until 8:00 p.m. which is way past my endurance level if I have been up most of the day. Back at the hotel, our night-time entertainment consisted of watching the baseball play-off game on television.

At daylight we were on the road home again. So much for

a vacation. One day traveling. One day recuperating from the journey. Another day traveling home. Next time we will plan better and certainly stay longer. Somebody gave me some good advice once: "If you are going to go cross-country skiing, start with a small country." I wish I had listened.

Oppie, our Chihuahua, and Mo Mo, our cat, welcomed us home enthusiastically. You would have thought we had been gone three months instead of three days. I hugged them, fed them and promptly went to bed. Buddy brought in the suitcases and climbed into bed also.

Ain't life exciting!

Journal Entry Twenty-three

I am shivering under two blankets. My fever is up. I am sneezing and ache all over. Flu season? Yes, but Beijing influenza isn't the reason for my symptoms. I am having side-effects of the chemotherapy that dripped into my chest port a couple days ago. For two hours the I.V. bag, thumb-tacked to the wall, delivered the paradoxic treatment. In order to get better, or to survive temporarily, I have to become sicker.

Every month, as long as I choose to endure it, I will have Chemojing flu. At least with this drug I will keep my hair and have limited nausea. In addition to the monthly infusion, I take a host of pills which have side-effects too. Then there are more pills to swallow to counteract those side-effects.

My oncologist upped my oxygen level one-third. She increased the time-released Morphine one-third. Yet, well-meaning folks tell me I look good. That statement is a pet-peeve of a lot of my metastatic friends. We don't know how to respond to it.

While we are glad we don't look like someone barely surviving in the jungles of the third world, we somehow feel our integrity is being challenged. Like we are being accused of somehow faking the disease. There have been times when I have wanted to display my x-rays to show people what is going on inside which they can't see. I have a notebook full of medical reports that aren't the least bit hopeful. The word *terminal* unavoidably sticks out, a reminder that this is a marathon life and death battle.

I wonder if ignorance would not have been more blissful. If I didn't know this was widely spread cancer, I would have thought the bone pain was arthritis. The breathing problems asthmatic. The low energy old age.

I cannot in good conscience just sit and wait for death. However, there are self-imposed limits as to how far I will go before compromising my fragile quality of life. Except on my worse days, with measured effort, I can still write some and teach my Sunday School class. This is my fifth year with the Builders

Class at McConnell Memorial. The class is very understanding as I port my oxygen tank to the front of the room, frequently sip water and occasionally make a dash to the restroom between lesson points.

When you get to this stage in life, the phoniness is gone. You are who you are, transparent to the soul. You may as well be. Everybody who knows you, or knows *of* you, is aware that you are the lady with cancer. Having a terminal disease is like having a huge, gray, dying pachyderm in the living room.

In one of Anne Landers' columns, Terry Kittering shared a similar comment: "There is an elephant in the room. It is large and squatting, so it is hard to get around it. Yet we squeeze by with 'How are you? 'And 'I'm fine'...and a thousand other forms of trivial chatter."

People seem to timidly dance around mortality. Death is inevitable regardless of the course we take. Dying, for me, isn't the primary issue. I am ready when He is. Death is the easy part. Living day to day in the here and now is much harder. I need some chicken soup.

Journal Entry Twenty-Four

Buddy left me last week. I will never be the same. In our nearly thirty-five years of marriage, we have seldom missed sharing the same bed at night. The few times we have been separated were mainly forced upon us. Mostly we were apart due to illness. While hospital beds aren't meant for sharing, often we have managed to snuggle side-by-side with the bed rails up. We are a two-some, period. Since the recurrence of cancer, Buddy has become ever-present, day and night. Sometimes that is a minor annoyance, but I know many women who would love to have my problem.

Buddy has a 97-year-old mother in Mississippi. Though reasonably healthy, his sister says she is beginning to wilt at a fast pace. At my insistence, Buddy went to visit her. After losing my own mother a year ago, I know how important those last visits are. I assured him I would be alright for a few days. I had plenty of oxygen on hand. My prescriptions were filled. Neighbors and friends were just a phone call away. Secretly I looked forward to being totally on my own for a few days.

Buddy was up at daylight on Tuesday. I fixed his coffee and made small talk while he double-checked his list. Flashlight. Vitamins. Shaving kit. Clothes. Money. With a kiss and a lingering wave, he was gone and I was alone. For the first couple of hours, I leisurely enjoyed the newspaper and watched the morning news. I felt totally unencumbered.

My mind raced as I thought about all I could accomplish in Buddy's absence. I had endless projects that require hours of concentration. I would finally have unlimited time to master a new digital camera, catalog my paperweight collection, plus install some computer programs that have been sitting around for months. Maybe I could even find time to outline a book. With Buddy constantly popping in and out of the bedroom and office, I can never find a sufficient span of time to indulge in long-term projects. You need to understand that Buddy has never been a loner. He has to have company to change a light bulb.

So here I was with five days before me. Other than my usual weekly responsibilities of writing a column and preparing a Sunday School lesson, I had 120 hours to do what I pleased.

Suddenly the power went out. No lights. No heat. No nothing. It was nearly noon and I needed electricity to accomplish the things on my list.

I sat and waited, hoping it was only a momentary glitch. No such luck. In the semi-darkness, I dressed and waited impatiently. Not wishing to waste the rest of the day, I got into the car and drove. All those interesting little shops I had always wanted to visit lured me. After dark, I arrived home totally exhausted with nobody to scold me for over-doing myself or to bring in my loot. Where was Buddy when I needed him?

The electricity was back on, but one turn of the faucet brought despair. The well pump was off. It always quits when the electricity does. Buddy had shown me years ago how to get the well pump pressure up again, but was I supposed to remember? No flushing toilets. No coffee water. Where was Buddy when I needed him?

I locked both outside doors and put on the chains. I bolted the bedroom door and climbed into bed. I wrapped myself around two pillows, pretending they were Buddy. I had hardly closed my eyes when I heard something fall in the kitchen. I remained awake the rest of the night watching the door and clutching a 38 magnum revolver. Where was Buddy when I needed him so I could sleep?

Two different couples invited me for supper. The food and fellowship was good, but the absence of Buddy's dry wit and growing-up tales was noticeable to me. I felt like a widow.

A friend invited me to lunch on Thursday. I waited over an hour for her to come. She never did. She forgot me. Buddy has never forgotten me. Never.

Sunday afternoon, I anxiously went to the door every thirty minutes. Buddy was due home anytime. It didn't matter that I had gotten nothing grand accomplished during those five days.

All I wanted was Buddy, my buddy.

Journal of a Living Lady

continues

Journal Entry Twenty-Five

This is a brief up-date. As I write this, I am literally sitting on the edge of my hospital bed using a pen and pad. I have been here nine-days following a sudden turn for the *not-so-good.* Instead of heading off to my brother's home and meeting up with my family for Thanksgiving, some are coming here. I am getting this brief respite from the hospital because neither patients nor doctors want to be on the premises for the next few days. So much for the holidays.

As I said before, terminal illness is a roller-coaster ride. Ups and downs. Dead stomps. Jump starts. This too shall pass.

Note from Editor:

In the newspaper business, deadlines tend to drive your week. You see the looming time crunch and the empty pages. If you have half the smarts you need, you'd better get on the move...and fast. The nature of this business allows for no slackards or whiners.

For months Nancy Kelly has been writing to deadline, many times from home, sometimes from a hospital bed. Hooked up by IV's and tethered by an inordinately short oxygen line, Nancy taps away on her laptop computer. Keeping her column going is a commitment one step below her Sunday School class preparation. She knows how important the "Living Lady" is to both readers ill themselves with cancer and those of us who have forgotten how to live fully.

I've felt a little "holier-than-thou" at times when I've beat a nasty deadline. Perhaps even a bit smug. But I get brought back down to earth real fast. There's a deadline I get reminded of each day, one which neither of us will ever beat.

But the real deadline isn't death. It's life.

We're all on a constant deadline. Most of the time we don't even realize it. Or a least act like it.

Nancy lives with a terminal gray elephant each day. She knows it's there. There's no shaking it. But I've never seen her scared. She has faith.

She has shared her life intimately with us. She's reminded me to have a little fun along the way, to keep things in perspective, not to be morbid about living and dying, to trust in God.

Nancy trusts in God completely. I've never asked her, but I suspect she thinks God has a sense of humor. After all, look at us.

When newspaper mania threatens to overtake me, Nancy helps get me on track. Without saying a word, she reminds me of the real deadlines we're all meeting. She's a good friend. She doesn't pull any punches. She takes me to task when I need it and cheers me on when I falter. I'm sure she's a better friend to me than I am to her.

I don't know when and how I'll die, at least not yet. But I do know that reading Nancy's columns has allowed me to live a little more deeply.

There not much more you can ask from a friend, is there?

Margit Blekfeld-Sztraky
Sentinel Editor

Journal Entry Twenty-Six

So much for patient privacy. Sitting in a hospital wheelchair waiting for my turn at the x-ray machine, I noticed the duct tape attached to the front of my chart. In huge letters was written, "Patient mildly hallucinatory last p.m." I groaned.

Hallucinatory? I guess I was hallucinating when the aides were hauling me out of my hospital room onto an ambulance stretcher to make a trip to another facility at 3:00 a.m.

Yes. 3:00 a.m.

Seems this hospital's open MRI was on the blink. Even when available, all the out-patients got the day spots. Now we in-patients were being carted off like human cargo to somewhere else in the middle of the night. Seemed unreal to me, but it happened.

"How much do you weigh?" the technician asked when we got to the other facility's radiology department. I begrudgingly gave the three-digit number in an undertone. The technician, surrounded by an entourage of strangers, announced my weight quite loudly to someone waiting in the isolation booth. I might have forgiven her if she had relayed it in kilograms. But no. She used pounds.

"Did you have to make a public announcement?" I asked disapprovingly as I laid strapped to the stretcher.

"Well, we are supposed to weigh you ourselves," she said, uncaring that I am sensitive about my weight even in the wee hours of the morning.

The idea of an open MRI is that you don't feel so confined. I confess to being extremely claustrophobic. The last open MRI I had at another hospital went fine because I could see sunshine and smell the fresh air. I was completely satisfied that I could escape the machine at any moment I wished.

This supposedly open MRI was more enclosed. It made me feel cooped. MRI is not an acronym for Merry Rider Incarcerated, but I tried to cooperate.

The technician came back. "We have to do it all over again. You moved." I rolled my eyes in dismay..

"You will have to let me sit up a few minutes, " I said, commenting honestly that this was not my idea of an open MRI machine. Out-of-sight, but within hearing range, I overheard the technician's comment to a co-worker that we had another one of those “deceptive". complainers.

The concrete-like tube moved down and I was assisted to an up-right position. Obviously I was causing a back-up in scheduling and they weren’t happy. Guess they were working on a deadline for me to be back to the original hospital before breakfast. Inquiring relatives might miss me and wonder if I was in the morgue.

Granted that night I was doped up. The sudden, excruciating pain from the cancer is what had originally sent me to the emergency room. But I knew where I was at 3:00 a.m. I knew Buddy had not known when he kissed me good-night that I would be miles away in a few hours. I didn't enjoy being treated with such indifference.

Finally the technicians got their pictures and I got another ambulance ride back to the first hospital. It was post-breakfast and I was just in time for my bone scan in the radiology department. There were certainly no delusions of grandeur in the austere hospital hallway. I was half-covered with a skimpy gown, sunken in a wheel chair and reading somebody's assessment of my mental state posted in bold letters.

Hallucinatory? Dream on.

Journal Entry Twenty-Seven

The most amazing fact about waking up each morning for me is that I am alive for another day. I am through asking how long I have. Even though doctors give educated guesses based on experience and statistics, in actuality, only God knows. It is not a major issue anymore as I've learned to be grateful for each day and not to take tomorrow for granted. All I ask is that my next of kin makes sure I am truly dead before burying my body. I have a reason for requesting this.

Even though I was born and raised in the South, I never understood the term "wake." Maybe it is a cultural thing. We had "viewings" and funerals, but the idea of sitting around with the body was not something my family did during my childhood. Since my parents and grandparents are all deceased now, I can't ask if it was a custom further back in our history.

Death has been a subject I've become accustomed to since the recurrence of my cancer. Curiosity got the best of me and I researched the word wake. What I discovered was quite interesting.

Seems that lead cups were formerly used to drink whiskey and moonshine. The combination of lead and alcohol often knocked the user out for a couple of days. Eventually someone would come along, take the person for dead, and prepare the body for possible burial. During the interim, the body was laid out on the kitchen table and the family would gather around, eating and drinking, waiting to see if the person would wake up. Hence the custom of holding a wake.

My grandfather, an O'Leary, was born in Ireland. He was raised in a London, England orphanage for a few years and was eventually adopted by a Canadian family named "White." Consequently, I have always had a personal interest in English history.

It seems that England developed a serious problem in the

late 1800's. This little country started running out of places to bury people.

Englanders would dig up coffins and take the bones to an undisclosed place to allow the reuse of the grave for a while. In the course of doing this, an eerie fact was uncovered. At least *one* out of every twenty-five caskets had scratch marks on the inside. Apparently the English had unknowingly been burying people alive.

This led to the idea of tying a string around the wrist of the deceased. The string would be threaded through the wooden coffin and up through to the exposed ground where it would be tied to a bell. This is where the term "graveyard shift" originated and other phrases liked "saved by the bell" and a "dead ringer."

To prevent a lot of wasted time, if my doctor says I am dead, check to see if I am breathing. If I am, hold a wake. If my chest is not going up and down, bury me. If you hear a bell, your oven timer just went off.

Journal Entry Twenty-Eight

Christmas Eve is my birthday. It has been a year and yet it seems like yesterday my sister was decorating the house and going all out to make it my best birthday ever. My mother always did that and now my sister, Sunnie Anne, believes in carrying on the tradition. She and one of my brothers will be coming from Memphis tomorrow night to do my birthday all over again. I think the theme this year will be "Fifty-five and still alive."

I am grateful for fifty-five years. Though I still feel young, I can now legitimately order off the senior menu at Shoney's and the IHOP. There are a few restaurants that still hold off discounts until the age of 62 or even 65, but we still benefit as Buddy passed those mileage marks a while back.

Now, when I am forgetful, maybe I can seriously plead a "senior moment." Either that or old-timer's disease. I read this week that there are many more mentally ill people than originally thought. In fact, the statistics on sanity are that one out of every four Americans is suffering from some form of mental illness. I thought of my three best friends and they are all okay. Hmm.

Time and tide wait for no sandcastle, no matter how well it is built. I still have hopes and dreams. If illness doesn't take me, old age probably will. I have had a good life in spite of this metastatic cancer.

I grew up poor in material things, but rich in the things that mattered. My family has always loved me and I have loved them. I had excellent teachers and acquired a good education. The best gift any teacher ever gave to me was the ability to read. It opened the world to this poor little girl who wanted to experience it all.

I have raised worms, spoken at universities, raised rabbits, been on national television, raised Great Danes, been a ventriloquist, raised exotic birds, flown airplanes, raised kittens, been on the front page of the Wall Street Journal, and raised guinea pigs.

The only thing I haven't done that I really wanted to do was sky dive. I had a knee replaced a few years ago and wouldn't attempt it now. Someday, when this life is over, I intend to sky rise though.

Birthdays never bothered me. Age doesn't matter unless you are cheese. These things I have learned in five and a half decades. Forget about the past. You can't change it. Forget about the future. You can't predict it. Forget about the present. I don't have you one. Merry Christmas anyway. It is the thought that counts.

Journal Entry Twenty-Nine

This is it, the new millennium. Maybe this is the century that the cure for cancer will be found. With all the money given for research, you would think that cancer would already be eradicated like Small Pox and Polio. It amazes me that so many people think that cancer is already licked. Not so, no matter what the media says. We have made a lot of progress and there is promising research. Yet, cancer is still the number two killer in America. Heart disease is number one.

Doctors told me months ago that I will never be cured of cancer. On a scale of one to four, four being the worst, I am Stage Four. This means the original cancer has spread (metastasized) to other body sites. In my case it went from the breast to the lungs, lymph system, and then to the bones. Stage four is considered terminal. There is no magic bullet for cancer. It is not a single disease. Cancer begins when a living cell goes for a wild ride with hundreds of other faulty genes. Sometimes it plays a cruel game of "hide and seek." There was a twelve year interval before my first diagnosis and its recurrence. The five-year mark is an oft-repeated myth.

This last year I have lost many friends to this disease. Most recently I attended the graveside service for Gary Hudson. He was in my Sunday School class and the same age as my husband, Buddy. Gary found out about his lung cancer the same month I found out about my recurrence of cancer. We e-mailed almost everyday, cheering each other on. We would use the telephone if a day or two went by without hearing from the other. We talked at great length about chemotherapy, radiation, and the pros and cons of surgery. We shared our cancer war stories and brief victories. When Gary began losing his thick hair, I offered him my wig.

We shared the same home nurse. Hospice would never acknowledge that either of us were patients because of patient privacy concerns. We found that policy amusing and purposely dropped each other's name to the nurse occasionally. She pretended not to hear or wouldn't comment.

Gary and I discussed life and death. Sometimes the conversations were light, but many times we honestly shared our concerns.

Neither of us wanted to leave our spouses alone. Both of us firmly believed II Corinthians 5:8 which greatly comforted us: *to be absent from the body* is to be present with the Lord. We wondered what that instantaneous step into eternity would be like. It must have been okay. When Gary drew his last breath, he smiled.

As Gary grew weaker and unsteady, I accused him of trying to beat me to heaven, never really believing he would. He did and I will miss him. Gary was an inspiration to all who knew him.

On Sunday, the day after Christmas, I stood arm and arm with his wife, Peggy. Members of Gary's family, as well as many mutual friends, stood silently on the windy hillside. We solemnly stared at the small, earthen cavity that would hold the canister of Gary's ashes. Along with our teary-eyed pastor, Dr. Rudy Patton, we quoted Psalm 23 and the Lord's Prayer. Brother Patton reminded us of Gary's valiant battle and his ever-present optimistic attitude.

My own burial plot is less than a hundred yards away from where we were standing. I couldn't help but think that this could have been me. That day the service was for Gary. Someday the funeral will be for me. Until then, I must keep on keeping on. If the situation had been reversed, that is what Gary would be doing.

Journal Entry Thirty

Until the horse is dead, I won't dismount. I only plan to spend the last day of my life dying. The rest of my days I intend to live life to its fullest.

Last Thanksgiving I was very, very sick. It was strange timing. This was the date that one of my doctors had given me as the latest estimate of my life expectancy. After all, I have metastatic cancer or do I? The doctors say I do. Pathology reports are explicit. However, as I write this I don't feel so sick or at least not sick unto death.

Wouldn't it be a statement to the reality of prayer if I lived another decade or so? Truthfully, I am making a statement to the reality of prayer just being here today.

Recently I went horseback riding in North Carolina. Everything was going fine until the horse started bouncing out of control. I tried with all my might to hang on, but was thrown off. Just when things could not possibly get worse, my foot got caught in the stirrup. When this happened, I fell head first to the ground. My head continued to bounce as the horse did not stop or even slow down. Just as I was losing consciousness, the Wal-Mart manager came and unplugged the horse. *Gotcha*

There are other important things that affect our mortality. I believe every survival kit should include a sense of humor. It is true that he who laughs *lasts*. Time flies whether you are having fun or not.

My 97-year-old mother-in-law is still a joy to be around. She has a strong Christian faith and laughs a lot. How fortunate I was to marry Buddy and get her in the deal.

Attitude is a big factor in how long we live. Attitude determines our altitude. I don't like being around pessimistic people. They depress me. I go out of my way to avoid negative people. Two negatives might make a plus in algebra, but not in life.

My lively grandmother always got the prize for the tackiest hat at the senior citizen party. She almost lived to be 100-years-old. I think it no coincidence that Grandma had a long life because she maintained a joyful, optimistic attitude. Each time, after she buried her husband, eight brothers and sisters and then four of her children, she grieved greatly, but briefly. Life then went on.

At times we take ourselves too seriously. Probably we would worry less about what people think of us if we knew how seldom they did. We aren't nearly as important as we sometimes think we are. Cemeteries are full of indispensable people.

Journal Entry Thirty-One

My first trip to the hospital this decade is now history. I survived the monthly round of chemotherapy in my oncologist's office with minimal difficulties. After three days, I felt invincible again. Like a normal woman, I was washing clothes and off to the grocery store. Like a foolish woman, I kept going. Pneumonia and flu took advantage of my vulnerability. In the middle of the night, a rasping cough and a raging fever put Buddy in a frenzy. He had me in the warmed up car before daybreak.

Buddy and my doctor have a mutual understanding to ignore my wishes. You need to understand I don't "volunteer" to go to a hospital.

The emergency room was full of cases like mine. Continual streams of coughing, wheezing, germ-laden patients were led into curtained cubicles. An old man, unshaven and shivering, was sitting in a wheel chair wrapped only in an afghan over boxer shorts. The whole emergency area had overtones of a plague.

When the emergency physician noted my complicated history, he told me I was in the worst place I could possibly be. He commented, with a twinkle in his eye, that he had sent his own mother home "to keep from killing her."

Six hours later, I was admitted. Six days later I wish I had stayed home. The weather had turned icy. It was the week-end and the hospital was noticeably understaffed.

Each day my fever returned. Dehydration became a problem. I vomited for what seemed like eternity. All my medications had to be changed to IV because I couldn't keep anything down. Patches were substituted for the morphine pills. However, there wasn't an intravenous substitute for one particular drug I routinely take, so a substitute medicine was ordered.

A weary nurse who had been on duty much too long appeared beside my bed with a pair of horse-size syringes. She said the medicine was to be pushed slowly into my porta-cath near my heart. That seemed like a huge dose to replace one aspirin size pill. Before I could express my concern, the respiration therapist interrupted by pulling a mask over my mouth for a breathing treatment. She quickly left the room for her next respiratory case. Talk about bad timing.

As the nurse began emptying the first syringe into my port, I tasted the drug and felt a fiery sensation of heat coursing through my body. I yelled at the nurse to stop. My chest was tightening. She look puzzled, but continued to push the syringe.

I flung the mask off my face and told her in no uncertain terms to stop NOW. She reluctantly did, but not before most of the first syringe had been emptied. My heart raced and I could have sworn that I felt the breath of angels.

To my disbelief, the nurse disappeared from the room. I was alone. My gut feeling was that I was experiencing a drug over-dose. In a panic, I ripped the narcotic patches off both arms and hurled them at the wastebasket in a desperate effort to stop the effects.

I then laid motionless, taking slow deep breaths in hopes that my heart would return to a normal rhythm. In a few minutes the nurse returned, flipping casually through a drug reaction book.

She scolded me for removing the patches. "We are supposed to return them to the dispensary." That nurse will never know how close she came to being plaster on the wall at that moment.

I have lived to fight cancer another day. But if I had died there in the hospital room, I am convinced nobody would have ever known the difference. Everyone would have always believed that I died from "complications of cancer."

Journal Entry Thirty-Two

Next week is Valentine's Day. Romantic cards, candy, and flowers arrangements beckon to be bought. You can't see the smug smile on my face. One year, during the early part of our marriage, Buddy forgot Valentine's Day. He never has since.

Being remembered on Sweetheart's Day was a given. To be forgotten on an anniversary or February 14th was the biggest mistake a husband could make.

Our first Valentine's Day after marriage consisted of a nice evening, complete with roses, cards, and a candle-lit dinner at a fancy restaurant. Our first anniversary was celebrated around the top layer of our wedding cake which had been frozen for twelve months. The second Valentine's Day was nice as was our second anniversary when Buddy gave me more roses and a beautiful, hand-picked card that I have in an album somewhere. But the third Valentine's Day. That was the occasion Buddy forgot.

I never hint at our anniversary or Valentine's Day simply because a reminder shouldn't be needed. April 24, 1965, should be forever etched in the circuitry of Buddy's brain. After all, he married me in a large church complete with two ministers and a huge reception attended by more people than anticipated. My Aunt Anne, who had catered the affair, had to send to the store to get more sherbet and ginger ale while we stood forever in the receiving line.

Buddy is by nature a shy fellow and his love for me was being seriously tested by all this attention. His most memorable comment, as we were on our way to our honeymoon in Bermuda, was that if he had known what all weddings involved, he would have eloped alone. I could have joined him later.

During his working years, Buddy was an airline mechanic, first for Pan Am Airlines, then Eastern Airlines, and finally Northwest Airlines. February, 1968 was a cold, snowy month in Memphis. He was then working the second shift glycoling airplanes, an important processes which keeps ice from forming on the wings. I was teaching first grade. Our working schedule conflicted and didn't allow for a lot of communication.

It was Valentine's Day, 1968. Of course, I had valentines on my mind. Who wouldn't with a class full of eager six-year-olds excitedly exchanging cards at the end of the day. I already had at least thirty cards, plus plenty of cupcakes and boxes of heart-shaped candy. But Buddy would be home after mid-night and I planned to be up waiting with candles lit on the dining table surrounding his favorite meal. I had just read a book about some silly romantic notion of meeting your husband at the door with just an apron on.

Midnight passed. No Buddy. One o'clock a.m. No Buddy. He could have at least called, I fumed. The candles burnt down. The meal was tossed out at three o'clock a.m. I was half worried and half mad. How could he forget Valentine's Day?

A few minutes later the front door creaked open. Snow frosted his heavy black eyebrows. "What are you doing still up?" he asked as he unloaded his heavy overcoat on the rack.

"Waiting on you," I said. "Where have you been?"

"Where do you think I have been?" he retorted. "Working my tail off in the freezing weather."

"You could have called."

"I tried to. The phones are out."

Buddy looked puzzled, not fully comprehending that my hair was fancier or that I had on red lipstick. He did notice the burned down candles on the table.

"Power been out here too?"

"Yes," I lied, feeling quite foolish. "Want some hot chocolate?"

"Not now. All I want to do is to go to bed."

I never mentioned Valentine Day that night. I put on my flannel pajamas and crawled into bed with him. Soon the alarm sounded and I headed off to school leaving Buddy in deep slumber. When I got home that afternoon, there was a note on the table.

"I'm sorry I forgot. Will make it up to you tonight." And he did.

Journal Entry Thirty-Three

This current Valentine Day is one I will never forget either. Generally, at our age, we just blurt out what we want for a special occasion. Hinting is for young folks who can still hear well.

I told Buddy no roses this year. For that price I could get something more touching like a therapeutic massage. With a son in college, luxuries are low on our priority list. I knew that this was a splurge request, but figured since Buddy would buy roses and take me to dinner anyway, it was a feasible substitute. Instead of eating out, I would treat him to his favorite meatloaf dinner with candlelight.

What Buddy requested for Valentine's Day surprised me. He has always wanted and I have always refused a pet pig. Not that we didn't have a baby pig once. We did. Buddy kept him in the back of our three acres in Stockbridge. Porky was an entertaining pet. He looked forward to Buddy's coming home from work each day and squealed and did a jig when he heard the old truck turn the corner. They played ball and "hide'n seek". Porky loved apples.

Alas, as all pigs do, Porky grew and grew and grew. Finally we had a 400 pound pet that was eating more than our family, including a host of needy kids who were living with us at the time. Our family could never have eaten Porky, so Buddy gave him to a co-worker who left singing, "This little piggy went to market." That mean man had Porky slaughtered the very next day and his family ate him all year. So much for the pig phase. At least I thought so.

But this Valentine Day, Buddy wanted a pet pig. Not a yard pig, but one to be kept in the house. Now I am an amiable person. But a pig in the house? That is really testing the limits of my congeniality.

Yet, Buddy is not your usual husband. He is kind, helpful, and loves me to a fault. Actually he is hard person to say *no* to.

Knowing that my days are considered numbered, I decided to let him have his pet pig as a parting present. I didn't tell him I was seriously trying to find a piglet. I just rolled my eyes anytime the subject came up.

A friend helped me locate a genuine pig farmer not too far from the house. I called the pig breeder who confirmed he had piggies all sizes. I told him I wanted a baby for my husband and would be by before Valentine to pick him up.

My sister was in town, so on Friday we shopped for the best, most expensive high protein pig pellets we could find. Next we got some good quality kitty litter and a huge paint roller box to serve as "Gussy's" litter box. I never believed for a minute a pig could be trained to use a kitty box, but the research said she would.

My energy level is very low, especially in the afternoon, so by the time we got Gussy's collar and other toys, I was ready to let Buddy in on the surprise. I sent him to unload the trunk full of pellets. When Buddy came back into the house, there was a smile on his face from ear to ear. He searched every room looking for the piglet. He was disappointed that I hadn't already gotten him. I explained that the pig farmer was supposed to be home the next afternoon and he could go with me to pick his piglet out. Buddy and our son, Charlie, had already changed Gussy's name to Bacon.

Later the next afternoon my sister was was having a blind date. I certainly wanted to be back in time to meet the gentleman. Buddy and I left for the pig farm at about four in the afternoon.

The man I had spoken to wasn't home and his elderly father insisted there weren't any babies. I insisted that he must be mistaken since his son had told me so. The elderly man told us to drive up to the pig pens and look for ourselves. We walked in muck past our ankles from one pig pen to another. There were hundreds of hogs, each pen as full as the next.

We spotted a sow that must have weighted 1000 pounds. As for a piglet, the smallest pig that we saw weighed more than me and, until recently, I shopped in the plus department.

The hog smell was *not* something you would find in a fine perfume shop. You could have collected that stench, put it in a gas bomb, and destroyed a large, unsuspecting nation. It took less than twenty minutes for Buddy to decide he didn't want a pig after all.

We thanked the old gentleman as we drove out and headed home for quick showers. Neither of us said a word as we rolled down the windows and breathed the wonderfully fresh mountain air.

I am not one to waste food though. The pellets mixed up well with the meat loaf.

Oink. Oink.

Journal of a Living Lady

continues

Journal Entry Thirty-Four

Decisions. Normally I can make them and move on. Sometimes I am forced to re-evaluate. I decided several months ago to forgo any further chemotherapy. Quality of life became more important than quantity of life. My oncologist told me that it was a now or never decision.

I have followed all the proper protocols in this battle with cancer. I had lung surgery. I had the rough chemo for months that caused me to be weak, nauseous and lose my hair. I also had radiation twice. After a while, I was eager to live the remainder of my life on my own terms without medical intrusion.

I did opt for Aredia which is a type of chemotherapy that fills in where the cancer has spread to the bone. Aredia isn't as toxic as the real chemotherapy. I also take Arimidex which is a hormonal treatment for breast cancer available for a few who, like me, test EST positive. In addition, I take a dozen or more pills to boost the immune system and control pain.

With treatment, the average length of life with metastatic cancer of my type is 18 months. I am now several months past that and, over-all, my quality of life has been good with a few exceptions.

Now I face the quality vs. quantity decision again and plan to talk with my oncologist this week. For those who don't know the whole story, I first found out I had breast cancer in the mid-1980's. I asked the Lord to let me live to see our son Charlie graduate from high school. Though the longevity prospects even then weren't good, I did see Charlie graduate from high school in 1998. He is now at Toccoa Falls Christian College and is taking a heavy load of hours because he wants to graduate in three years rather than four. He hopes that I will be around at least long enough to see him get that important sheep-skin. He is now only 15 months away from graduation. I never strongly felt my seeing Charlie graduate from college was a realistic goal though I have maintained hope and faith. God has sustained me thus far to everybody's amazement. It is certainly within his sovereign power to continue to do so.

Though there are never any guarantees, in order to "buy" fifteen months probably means I will need to undergo the more drastic chemo once again. Am I ready to lose my hair? Am I ready to puke for days at a time? Am I ready to be pushed in a wheelchair because of the resulting neuropathy?

Do I want to see Charlie graduate from college? You bet! If he can make the sacrifices with the extra studies, work twelve hours on Saturdays, spend precious time with me on Sundays after church, I am willing to give it my best shot.

Just pray it is not too late.

Journal Entry Thirty-Five

Last week I told you my about my current dilemma in choosing quality of life over quantity. I decided several months ago to go for quality for whatever time I had remaining with metastatic breast cancer. At the time it was the right choice.

I did choose to remain on light chemotherapy, a little radiation and some pills to keep me functional for as long as possible without losing too many good days. I don't regret the decision as I have had several decent months. This has enabled me to continue writing this column without interruption and has allowed me to continue teaching my adult Sunday School class. I can only do that when my mind is relatively clear and I have a normal amount of energy for at least part of the day.

Unfortunately my health has been declining for several weeks. Subtle changes in weight, stumbling and weakness have become more noticeable.

Because Charlie's graduation from college is getting closer, my decision has changed. While I would still like to have quality of life, I am willing to endure the side-effect and indignities of aggressive cancer treatment if it means I might can make it long enough to see Charlie get that diploma.

I asked that you pray that it wasn't too late to slow the course of this disease. While there aren't any guarantees, my doctor believes it is worth the try and didn't waste any precious time getting started. I just completed six hours of chemotherapy.

My oncologist has encouraged to set some short-term goals. She has encouraged me to travel while I am able. If money weren't an issue, there are quite a few places I would like to visit, but if I never get to those places, it is okay.

I have gotten wonderful cards and e-mail from readers. I rarely share them because my mama taught me not to stretch my arms patting myself on the back. That is not my intention now. However, I feel compelled to relate the following.

Several months ago, a man and his wife, total strangers, drove from Alabama to visit me in the hospital on a day when I was very sick. I tried to be hospitable and cheerful, but frankly was having a difficult time of it.

This man sent me an e-mail recently after reading my latest column. I only share it with you so you can know how God uses the encouragement of strangers, friends, and family to keep me going and to give wisdom just when I need it.

He said, "*...I don't feel the pain and the nausea and weakness and the hopelessness/futility of a painful drive down a dead-end street, but I need to tell you in all honesty that your journals are an on-going inspiration to me. There is simply no way that you or I can even assess on this side of Glory the impact they will have on eternity.*

'My real opinion, dear friend: that impact will be more than worth whatever pain is required of you to carry on until God closes the door that no man can open. The ones which so eloquently tell of pain with humor are precisely the ones which show me the most of the grace of God. It would grieve me to think I might contribute in any way to your pains, but I really, really do have to be honest and tell you how much your journals mean to me and, no doubt, to others.

'It is natural to be unassuming and not take credit for a positive spiritual impact on eternity, but please, dear lady, do recognize the Spiritual Gift that GOD has given you which is weekly building the kingdom of our Lord here and in eternity, though your exercise of that gift through your journals..."

Bob Cleveland

That I could be a blessing to others through this illness makes it worthwhile. Thank you, Bob, and to others who encourage me and make me smile, though sometimes through tears.

Someone else wrote, in jest I hope: "My fingers are crossed, my legs are twisted into a knot. I will not eat until you are doing well."

I wrote back: "All is well, my friend. Get on with your life."

Journal Entry Thirty-Six

It was a first for me. I gave a eulogy recently for a good friend I never met. Her name was Carol. You would have liked her. I loved her. She was everything a good friend should be...loyal, loving, encouraging and a beacon of faith no matter how dark the shadows fell. She instinctively knew when it was appropriate to laugh, which she did often, and when it was helpful to cry. She, too, had metastatic cancer. We were sisters together on a shared pathway.

Carol and I met via the Internet in a world-wide, on-line community referred to as a "list." Carol and I, along with a few others, decided we needed a smaller, more intimate list specifically for those of us with metastatic breast cancer.

Club Mets was formed and right away we became a virtual sisterhood with a few male members who had breast cancer themselves or were care givers. By way of e-mail that all invited members could read, we could and did chat about most anything relative to the disease. Most importantly we were able to relate feelings and emotions that only those going through the fire could really understand. On any given day, somebody was going through a crisis. Anonymity was important. Only with permission would any of those comments be shared outside this close circle of cyber friends. We shared our lows and highs as well as fears.

Carol was the Club Mets cheer-leader. When somebody new joined the group, she enthusiastically welcomed them to the club nobody wanted to be a member of, yet was glad existed. It was a daily life-line.

Carol and I hit it off so well because we had so much in common. Both of us had breast cancer that had metastasized to the lungs and other areas. We both had loving husbands as caretakers and we both had sons. Carol and I were from the same state.

The two of us had been through the medical mill with

similar surgeries, chemotherapy and radiation. She and I preferred quality of life over quantity if that was the choice. The bond that held us together most was a mutual faith in the same Lord. Carol was a real Christian.

We were always making plans to meet for lunch at Town Center Mall with her husband, Lee, and my husband, Buddy. I am sorry we never did. Around November Carol took a bad turn. She wrote me: "*I am so struck by the sudden nature of my decline/demise. Sure, I knew it was coming, but was like water breaking over a dam when it did.*"

A month later she wrote again: "*The past several weeks have been unbelievable. They have whizzed by with surprisingly little memory for dates or sequence of events. They have been physically and emotionally grueling beyond anything I could image. There were booby traps, great disappointment, terrible surprises and news, fear. Yet, I have also experienced and felt the true meaning of love from my God, my husband, son, family, list friends, and little pets who stand guard over me.*"

When we talked on the phone, Carol never wanted to talk about Carol. She wanted to know how I was doing. The frailty of her voice conveyed to me that she was losing the battle.

Carol's final note to me said, "*I have lost track of time. My life and time is in God's hands. I know He will bring good out of this in His own way.*"

At the funeral, her gracious husband accompanied me to the casket. Carol, with her gorgeous long red hair, looked just like the pictures she had sent.

At the young age of fifty-two she had preached her own funeral. Yet tradition required a final service. Lee, as well as an ex-husband from younger years, a son, a sister, and several work friends spoke nothing but praise for Carol. The personal stories evoked both laughter and tears.

With assistance from Lee, I tottered to the front and spoke about my unusual relationship with Carol. Had I known that I would be asked to share the eulogy, I might have dressed up a bit more. With my bald head and the portable oxygen machine making pulsating noises, I related the best I could what an inspiration Carol had been to me.

In this journey of life it is how we live the dash between our birth and death dates that matters most. Carol was a shining example of not only how to live the dash but also how to finish the race with dignity and respect.

Journal

of a

Living Lady

continues

Journal Entry Thirty-Seven

This has been the most hectic week. We had a yard sale on Friday and Saturday. What work! We had boxes stored in the attic that haven't been opened since our move in 1994. Of course, I wasn't able to move boxes, but I did try to help sort through things and price the various items. It was obvious from the ragged newspaper and droppings that rats had been living rent-free in the boxes from the old barn. What free-loaders.

The day before the sale, we had three people arrive early. I am not one to turn down good money, so I made some sales and hoped that this would be a sign of prosperity for the next couple of days.

That same day I sold an advertised World War II German luger taken from an S.S. officer. A few years ago I had traded a nice set of commemorative coins for it. The actual buyer dickered a bit and in the end he bargained me down $50 from my original $300 asking price.

Three consecutive men came later in the day to see the vintage gun. Each insinuated that I had been robbed. One young man with a rusty old truck and two babies on the front seat said he had come expecting to pay $600.

Oh, well. Mistakes are the cost of education sometimes.

Before I had my first cup of coffee on Friday, ten people were on the front porch inspecting the used merchandise. Now I expect people to haggle a little at a yard sale, but some were really jerks.

“What will you take for this old pottery jug?"

Thinking that surely it was marked, I asked her what I had on it.

“It says $10," she answered.

“I'll take $8," I replied. "No less."

“I'll give you $6."

“No, $8 is as low as I'll go."

The lady put the jug down. Next she picked up a cast iron skillet that was marked $6.

"Will you take $3 for this?"

"No, but I'll take $5." She put the skillet down.

Finally she picked up the dulcimer that was well worth the $15 that was marked on it. "Will you take $7 for this music thing?"

"No, but I'll take $12." The lady headed down the steps without buying anything. I felt like bopping her on the head with that iron skillet. With my Christian up-bringing, killing wasn't an option. But it was a slow-fleeing thought.

Journal Entry Thirty-Eight

Everybody wants to know about the Oprah show. Frankly I am amused by the reaction of my family and friends. You would think I had just struck gold. Oprah is just Oprah. I am not one bit richer or poorer by meeting her though she was very nice and it was an interesting experience. Years ago I might have been star-struck, but cancer has a way of changing your values.

This Oprah saga started several days ago when, out of the blue, I got a phone call from an associate producer named Kelly of Harpo Productions. She asked me about my experience with the Making Memories Organization. This is the group that chose me for their first wish- granting opportunity late last summer. I had made a three sentence request on the Internet for a family reunion, never believing anything would come from it. After all, there are millions of people with cancer and who wouldn't want a wish granted?

Making Memories is a first-class, non-profit organization that grants wishes to metastatic breast cancer patients who usually have little funds for personal pleasures after the expenses of fighting the disease. Fran Hansen, the Executive Director, began the organization after having a cancer scare herself.

After explaining to the producer about the wonderful reunion we had at Brasstown Valley Resort and what a legacy of memories it had given my entire family, Kelly thanked me for the information. I thought that was that.

Within hours, she had phoned me three times. During the last call Kelly told me that Harpo was sending a team to our home the next day. She instructed me to gather all the videos, albums and news clippings I could get my hands on documenting my life, past and present.

It couldn't have been worse timing. We were in the middle of a yard sale and our lawn and porch looked like a front for the Salvation Army Thrift Store. I felt like laughing and crying at the same time. How surreal that national television was coming to our house in less than twenty-four hours.

This terminally ill lady came alive. You have heard of fur flying. Every particle of dust in the house was begging for a chance to get out of Lady Fuzzbuster's way. General Patton would have been proud of me, the way I organized Buddy. Then another call came.

"We have changed our minds," Kelly said. "We aren't coming tomorrow. We are sending a network courier to your house at 8:00 p.m. tonight to pick up your collection. We want to fly you to Chicago on Wednesday to be on the show. Can you travel?"

"Sure," I said, not thinking about little matters like carrying an oxygen tank on the airplane, walking more than a few feet without a wheel chair, plus the fact my bald head looked like a shiny pink bowling ball.

It all worked out. The next morning I taught Sunday School while a friend videoed it for possible inclusion on the show. Monday and Tuesday were a blur and our phone rung repeatedly as the word spread. On Wednesday morning, Buddy kissed me good-bye and waved sympathetically to my sister who flew in from Memphis to accompany me to Chicago. Buddy would have gone if I had insisted, but we didn't have a suitcase big enough to carry all the Pepto-Bismol we would need for this country boy who hates the limelight. When Sunnie Anne volunteered to go in his place, you would have though he had gotten a stay of execution.

I returned on Mother's Day week-end and we drove from the Atlanta airport to Mississippi to visit Buddy's 97-year-old mother. Ironically, she lives in the same town where Oprah was raised.

During the car ride home I developed pleurisy. The next morning I had my re-scheduled chemotherapy. It was back to the real world of battling cancer. No more riding around in chauffeured limousines longer than a Chicago block or staying in $400 a night hotels with an extra phone by the toilet. Yet, it was fun while it lasted.

Journal Entry Thirty-Nine

What happened to spring? My two favorite seasons of the year, spring and fall, seem to pass so quickly. I equally detest sizzling summers and frigid winters. Both are an endurance test for me.

A few years ago there was a classified ad in the Atlanta paper from a lady who wanted to escape the harsh Michigan winters. She was a widow and offered to help out around the house in exchange for room and board. At that time our boys were about ten-years-old. No, we don't have twins. We adopted our last foster child who is five months younger than Charlie.

I was working as a school principal and Buddy was still with the airlines. Having some domestic help and giving companionship to a lonely lady appeared to be a "win-win" situation. We even had a modest two-room apartment attached to the garage.

I wrote Lily Jean and learned that she had been married for over forty years to a union laborer and had been a stay-at-home mother and wife. Her children were all grown and she didn't want to be stuck indoors for another dreary northern winter.

She accepted our invitation to stay for three months. The day finally came for us to pick up our guest at the airport. The boys were excited, but Buddy and I were apprehensive as we carefully studied each woman as they came into the terminal. We held a picture of a petite lady who appeared to be in her late sixties. Lily Jean was the last passenger to disembark the plane and appeared anxious. When we introduced ourselves, she let out a high-pitched squeal of relief, happy that this wasn't a hoax.

We learned much about Lily Jean over the next few weeks. She had never learned to drive, but was a serious walker. Though we offered to drive her anywhere she wanted to go, she seldom took us up on it. Almost daily Lily Jean would walk for miles, stopping to chat with willing neighbors in our sprawling metropolitan suburb. Eventually she conversed with more people in our community than we had in over twenty years.

Lily Jean also enjoyed riding a bicycle. Buddy unhooked my fifty-ish Schwinn which had been hanging for years in the garage. He removed the cobwebs, replaced a rotting tire, greased the gears, added a mirror and finally a red horn. Lily Jean became quite an attraction as she leisurely rode in the neighborhood tooting her ooga-horn while waving a tiny American flag.

Lily Jean loved attending the Heart-to-Heart Sunday School class I taught. She made new friends quickly. Though she had never been a serious church goer before, Lily Jean adored our young pastor and listened to his tapes over and over. Before going home to Michigan, she was baptized one sunny Lord's Day.

There was only one blight during her visit with us. Lily Jean and Buddy had differences concerning the discipline of our boys whom she spoiled. When he asked her to refrain from taking up for the boys when he corrected them, it hurt her feelings. She never did warm up to Buddy again. In her sight, Mr. Kelly was like a harsh winter, to be *endured*. I was clearly her favorite.

Try as I might, I never could get Lily Jean to call me "Nancy." It was always, "Dr. Kelly," this and that, a title I don't encourage, though a few old colleagues and students still refer to me that way. She always put me on a pedestal I didn't deserve and sometimes embarrassed me by exaggerating my personal qualities to others. When she started wearing a large button with my picture glued to the front, I had to tell her what a poor, wretched creature I really was, though I am not sure she ever believed it.

We have kept in touch occasionally. Last year Lily Jean sadly wrote that she had been disappointed in love. I wondered how any suitor could spurn Lily Jean, that beautiful flower in my life who appeared for such a short season.

Journal Entry Forty

Yesterday was Buddy's sixty-eighth birthday. A childhood friend telephoned early in the morning to offer his condolences. My husband would need them before the day was over.

Other friends and relatives called. The postman personally delivered some nice cards. Charlie and I sang Happy Birthday around a cake with flaming candles. We gave him his gifts, including a hilarious, singing fish from my sister. Charlie gave him a beautifully framed poster. Besides clothes, I gave him a fly rod and accompanying gear in hopes that he would go fishing more often. Every man needs the solitude of throwing a line in the water and listening to the crickets crick. No clocks. No women. Nothing but man and nature.

Buddy spent most of his birthday working on screening our front port, a project he began a few days earlier. By late afternoon, he was tired and flopped into his recliner. When he started to untie his shoes, he felt severe indigestion-type pain. His heart started racing wildly.

A similar experience happened a couple of years ago when he was out walking. A lady at a restaurant called me. She told me Buddy was sitting on the curb in a daze. That time the emergency room doctor stopped Buddy's racing heart by giving him an injection. In a few minutes his heart was beating normally and we went home an hour or so later.

Buddy has since had several normal cardiograms and a negative stress test. Just recently he had a complete physical with no problems other than a mildly elevated cholesterol level. Buddy is a worrier though. My cancer always weighs heavy on his mind, but so do many other things like the humidity index and the national debt.

When Buddy called out to me from the recliner, I didn't hear him at first. He calls my name quite frequently in a day's time, so we have an understanding that if he ever really needs me, he is to call emphatically. The urgency in his voice let me know that I needed to immediately stop what I was doing.

Buddy told me to put my hand over his chest and feel the fast pounding. At that moment, the singing fish started blaring, "Don't worry. Be happy." I snatched the plug out of the wall.

"Do you want to go to the hospital?" I asked.

"Yes," he answered without hesitation.

"Okay. Ambulance or car?"

"Car," he replied.

I went to the door and called for Charlie. No answer. He was still jogging. Not a neighbor was in sight. It was just me and Buddy. I mumbled a prayer as I helped him to the car. The trip wasn't going to be easy. Buddy was understandably up-tight.

"Don't drive like an old lady," he complained, even though I was going 60 mph. I turned on the hazard lights and sped up a little, honking and passing traffic all the way to the hospital.

"My husband is having chest pains," I announced at the emergency desk. I fished Buddy's back pocket for his billfold with his insurance card. A nurse led him away through the double doors. After signing endless forms, I called the answering machine to leave a message for Charlie.

In the examining room, Buddy was hooked up to monitors. A nursing assistant was asking the routine questions. She turned around to tell me a PA was "on call." This news was not very comforting, but thankfully Buddy was better now. His blood pressure was good and his pulse was slower. The PA eventually arrived and ordered an EKG and blood work. They were normal also.

Charlie arrived just as we were leaving and was, of course, relieved to learn his Dad was alright. I wasn't going to be a widow that day nor was he to be suddenly fatherless. We both were genuinely grateful.

This was much ado about nothing perhaps, but a birthday Buddy will not forget. Now, if I can just get him to go fishing.

Journal Entry Forty-One

Some things are impossible like stuffing an elephant in a thimble or rounding off infinity. I've not tried either of these, but I have tried to lose weight. Impossible for me, at least for the long haul.

I have lost 200 pounds in my lifetime. Unfortunately, I've re-discovered every single fat module. I admit to having *elbow benditis* in the past. However, since having the cancer recurrence, I really and truly do not eat that much

My oncologist told me not to even think about dieting. She doesn't want me to lose any weight, though I have dropped about twenty pounds in the last year. I think she considers my weight like blubber on a bear, good for the survival mode during hard times. She is even giving me medicine to increase my appetite. That is a first.

My last serious attempt at losing weight came a few years ago. I was the assistant principal of a school and the administrator challenged me to a weight-loss duel. Both of us were much too heavy and each of us was extremely competitive. I am somewhat mellower now and hopefully have my values in order.

In those days I would rather die than lose a competition of any sort. Call it pride, perfectionism, or whatever. It was a contest of wills between Herb and me. Type A against Type A. The prize for the most weight loss during the twelve week period was $200, but it didn't matter. We would have battled for nothing.

Every week was weigh-in time in a little storage room at the school. Some of the teachers participated in the contest, but it was obvious from week one that it was going to be an ultimate duel between the administrators.

Herb went from double whoppers and french fries to lettuce, lean meat and water. I ate skinny sandwiches and walked around the parking lot twenty times during the lunch period. The first week we tied at a 7 pound loss. We congratulated each other, secretly believing next week would be different. The following week I had lost 4 pounds and Herb lost 3. We kept a huge graph near the office for all to see. That was quite an incentive for both of us. We continually see-sawed for top honors. The week before the final weigh-in found me down 46 pounds and Herb down 47.

Herb emptied his pockets each Friday before weighing. I noticed he wore light-weight clothing on weigh-in days. I didn't have any pockets to empty. However, when it was my turn, I took my shoes and stockings off and stood on my tip-toes, leaning on the scales to my advantage.

The night before the final weigh-in was a stressful, no-sleeper. Now mind you, this was a desperate situation. Desperate people do desperate things. Winning a war, any war, takes strategy and determination. I dug through the medicine cabinet and found some old diuretic pills, more commonly called water pills. Just one tiny white tablet kept me trudging endlessly during the night to the bathroom.

The next day Herb weighed in first. He shed exactly 3 pounds for a total of 50. After hearing the news, I snuck in the store room and weighed myself privately. Pooh! I had only lost 3 pounds for a total of 49. In my mind, I pictured the victory celebration for Herb. I would be the meek loser, obliged to congratulate the winner. Self-pity struck. All that starvation and then to lose by one pound. No way.

It was one of the most unscrupulous things I have ever done. Having had breast cancer surgery in 1986, I required a prosthesis for esthetic balance. So, with nobody looking, I removed that wobbly piece of pink plastic and stuck it in the drawer with the construction paper. I rationalized that it wasn't cheating. After all, it wasn't part of my original equipment.

After the monitor completed my official weigh-in, she announced that I had lost 4 pounds. It was a tie. Everybody was happy, including Herb and me. Neither of us had lost face. We shared the prize money and lived happily ever after.

Not really. I am sending him this column as a way of confession. He really won. I lost.

Journal Entry Forty-Two

Buddy's trip to the emergency room on his birthday is a hard act to follow. But I tried. Sunday afternoon I had shoulder pain like crazy. It wouldn't go away no matter what I took. Because of the cancer, I have an arsenal of pain killers available, but not even morphine helped. I thought, wimpy me. I can't even stand arthritis pain anymore. Where was the Nancy of old who hardly winced at needles or broken bones, the one who'd rather suffer all day than take an aspirin. Well, apparently she doesn't exist anymore. The pain was horrendous. Still I did not tell Buddy. He didn't need anything else to worry about with the national debt and all.

After retiring for the night, the shoulder pain improved some, but then I had chest pain. It was sort of like bad indigestion, only I seldom get anything as common as indigestion. I waited futilely for the elephant in my chest to come bursting through.

With Buddy snoring blissfully, I slipped out of bed and phoned the 24-hour "nurse on call," provided by my PPO insurance plan. After explaining the symptoms, she told me to go immediately to the closest emergency room. That wasn't what I wanted to hear.

I went back into the bedroom, flipped on the overhead light and announced to Buddy that he needed to take me to the ER. He was caught totally off-guard. He fumbled around for his shoes and socks while I waited somewhat impatiently for him to get his act together.

We went to a different hospital than the one where Buddy went on his ER trip. He announced at the desk that I was having chest pains and off I went through the ominous swinging doors. The staff couldn't have been nicer. The ER doctor asked the routine questions, ordered tests and a cardiogram. The nurse kept poking little white nitroglycerin pills down me and eventually the pain lessened to a mere annoyance. At 2:00 a.m., the hospital staff admitted me.

How unfair. Buddy got to go home. But, me, with a medical history that rivals War and Peace in volume, I am too risky to turn loose so quickly.

For whatever reason, I was given the best room in the hospital. They call it the "VIP" room. The admissions clerk must have checked with the ambulance services to be sure there weren't any real VIP's en route. I felt honored to have three wall hangings to stare at, a TV with a remote control that worked, plus a private bathroom with gleaming fixtures and even a sit-down shower stall.

We still don't know for sure what caused the pain, my heart or the cancer. Maybe it was a case of much ado about nothing. Hope so. I was sprung late the next afternoon.

Journal Entry Forty-Three

I don't know if the corpse was male or female. Nor do I know the color or age of the deceased. The funeral procession, consisting of a sheriff's car, a hearse and approximately twenty other cars, was slowly approaching. I signaled, pulled my car over to the far right edge of the highway and turned off the key.

Four teenagers in the car behind me didn't appreciate my gesture of respect. Perhaps they didn't know it is a southern custom to pull over when a funeral entourage is passing. It used to be the law. Regardless, it is still good manners.

Barely braking, the young driver stomped the gas pedal and rushed past my waiting car. A boy on the passenger's side relayed the driver's disgust by giving me a middle-finger salute. That punky kid doesn't know how lucky he was that Buddy wasn't with me. He wouldn't put up with anybody disrespecting a lady, particularly *his*.

A couple of years ago our family was leading the funeral procession for my mother. The Memphis traffic was heavy. It was one of the saddest days of our lives. My youngest brother, Bob, pointed out that several cars were pulling over to the curb. Grateful tears stained our cheeks. What a compassionate demonstration of respect for an unknown person who happened to be someone's daughter, wife, mother and friend.

In contrast, those teenagers who sped past the line of cars with their headlights on showed both their ignorance and arrogance. Sooner or later, death will visit their families. I suspect that only then will they realize the significance of this small act of kindness.

A funeral procession brings us face-to-face with universal reality. All the bad one can do in this life will have been done. All the good also. The Shakespearian lines I memorized in high school quickly come to mind. Regarding Julius Caesar, Anthony aptly said, "*I come to bury Caesar, not to praise him. The evil that men do lives after them; The good is oft interred with their bones;*

So let it be with Caesar. "

So it is with us. While we are yet living, we are writing our own eulogy. A candle loses no power by lighting another. May each of us spark a little light in this dark world.

And, to you, rude teenage boys. Someday when you are riding in the family car on the way to the local cemetery, I hope a hurried stranger will stop long enough for you to recognize and appreciate a traditional expression of sympathy.

Journal Entry Forty-Four

Buddy is a low-key, dry wit comedian. One of his expressions of mock self-righteous offense is, "Well, I never..." He throws his neck back, raises his eyebrows and tilts his nose upwards. It always bows me over with laughter.

The word *never* is one of those absolutes you can't quibble with. Yesterday I was pondering things I have never done, not that they are necessarily regrettable.

Not ever or at any time have I drunk whiskey. While there are other reasons I am a tee-totaler, I understand that whiskey is highly concentrated with calories. I have imbibed enough zero-caloried diet colas in my lifetime to fill the town's water tank. Ironically, my few whiskey-drinking acquaintances are skinny rails. I am as plump as a Georgia peach on Miracle-Gro. Go figure.

I have never jumped from an airplane though I have piloted several. My piloting expertise is definitely in the air and not on the ground. One fall morning I taxied a Cessna into a telephone pole. The worst part was calling Buddy to explain how I accomplished this amazing feat.

I have never been on a lobster-trapping vessel, but got up once at 3:00 a.m. to go bass fishing with my daddy in a tiny, patched-up wooden boat. He had three sons, but he chose me that day.

I have never seen a stack of million dollar bills, but neither have I begged for bread or lacked for a warm bed.

The nevers for me are never-ending.

I have never walked on the moon or been mugged on earth.

I have never been to Ethiopia or New Zealand, but have been to Israel, Mexico, Bermuda, Italy and Kosciusko, Mississippi.

I never heard an unkind word from my grandmother.

I have never been bitten by a snake, but when I was twelve, my mischievous older brother chased me all over the house with a huge, wiggly, rubber black moccasin. My heart has never been the same since.

I never pay retail or cry uncle.

Guess I am the Queen of Never-Never Land until the 12th of Never. Nevertheless and never more of this never-ending nonsense.

Journal Entry Forty-Five

As of my last medical report, I am stable. Stable is a good word when you have serious cancer. Sure I have bad days now and then, but don't we all? My hair is getting a tad longer and as curly as that of a Scottie dog. I only got called *sir* twice last week.

It is hard to know whether the pain in certain joints is the bone cancer surging or my nemesis, Arthur I. Tis. Some days I feel like wearing my right arm in a sling or grabbing my cane to walk, but most of the time I won't. I don't like the unnecessary attention. Occasionally I must carry my portable oxygen tank in public which I detest, but all in all, I am doing good for the shape I am in.

I have two weeks before more chemotherapy, so I am trying to figure out what to do in this hot weather. Our good friends sold their pontoon boat. Nobody else has invited us boating, so I am land-bound. We briefly had a jet ski, but Buddy sold it before I ever got a chance to try it out. I think he was afraid I would fall off and he would never get me back to shore. He was probably right, but don't tell him.

Not many summers ago, Buddy and Charlie were pulling me behind an old boat in an inner tube. My body came out of the snug tube. Don't ask me how. I couldn't get back into it or muster enough strength to pull myself into the boat. Buddy and Charlie tried to pull me out of the water, but my wet arms kept slipping out of their hands. It was a predicament for sure.

Finally, Charlie extended the boat paddle which I held onto while Buddy slowly idled the boat more than a mile to the concrete exit ramp. I *walked* out of the lake.

For some reason that inner tube is nowhere to be found now. Buddy has not been inclined to get me another one, but that is okay.

I smugly remember October, 1964. Those were our courting days. Buddy and I had gone out in a little boat on a lake not far from my home in Memphis. For some reason, we decided to swap ends. In the middle of the transfer, we spontaneously embraced and kissed. The boat capsized. My daddy wasn't too thrilled with Buddy or me when we arrived home after dark, soaking wet and shivering.

In spite of our water unworthiness, this goose married that gander and we are still floating.

Journal Entry Forty-Six

We have slowly accumulated a farm menagerie. Currently it includes four guineas, a pair of pygmy goats, two ducks, eight hens and a rip-roaring rooster. He is quite a braggart. Every time one of those hens lays an egg, which is quite often, he rises on his tiptoes and crows. By the end of the day that rooster is so lame and hoarse he needs crutches and throat spray. Buddy has offered to put him out of his misery, but I hid the shotgun.

I grew up in the city, but always wanted to live on a farm. Strange how many people I have met who grew up on a farm and always wanted to live in the city. Maybe we got switched at birth.

When I was nine, I decided to grow a garden in our crudely fenced backyard. I hoed an area about nine foot by nine. The neighborhood grocery store had a seed section, so I emptied my piggy bank and bought some butterbeans and corn. Sure enough, the seeds sprouted during that hot summer.

About that same time I fell in love with two little ducklings at the corner feed store. If I was going to be a bona fide farm girl, animals were a must. My parents didn't care as long as I took care of them. No problem. I snuck a pan out of mama's cupboard for water and fed the ducks scraps from the supper table.

Alas. A few days later I discovered all my hardy plants had vanished. I was bewildered and disgusted. Dying I could understand, but totally disappearing! How could that have happened?

Henry, a somewhat retarded twelve-year-old who lived behind us, said the ducks did it. I figured he must have heard his grandmother say that.

Nonetheless, the two ducks were definitely suspect. But the *death penalty*. Now that was too drastic no matter how disappointed I was in them. This is what happened.

The next week I went outside to play with Quacky and

Dacky. There they were, lying on the ground, deader than dirt. I screamed in anguish. The neighbors came running. Nobody could understand how those two full grown ducks could have just keeled over like that, their heads twisted to the side.

The next morning I answered a knock at the door. To my surprise stood Henry and his mother. Henry meekly handed me $5. His mother explained that it was he who had wrenched the ducks' necks. I was speechless.

My mama overheard Henry's sincere, but obviously practiced apology and eased into the living room. She gave Henry's mother a sympathetic look and lightly squeezed my shoulder. Taking her cue, I babbled that is was okay and that I'd get more ducks someday.

Henry was strange and I knew it, but he was usually such a gentle soul. I didn't sleep well for nights wondering what must have been in Henry's mind to do such a terrible thing. Now I understand that it was his form of justice.

Our present farm menagerie, including Quacky and Dacky II, reminds me of those childhood days of long past. We don't have a neighbor named Henry, but I am keeping my eye on Buddy.

Journal Entry Forty-Seven

I had begun another column that was supposed to run today, an amusing one. Yet, after a frank discussion with my oncologist this morning, a humorous column didn't fit my mood. My funny bone fractured with the news that the cancer has returned with a vengeance.

My shoulder has been aching for several weeks, yet I couldn't remember injuring it. I tried putting my arm in different positions in bed. No relief. I even exercised it with some light tree trimming thinking the painful kink would work out. It didn't.

Last week I discovered an egg-shaped lump deeply embedded under my right arm. It seemed oddly familiar, like the one I found in 1984, just before the original diagnosis of breast cancer. There was twelve year interval between that first surgery and the recurrence of cancer in 1997 which invaded my lungs and back. After a downward spiral, including a stint with hospice, I miraculously bounced back to near normalcy in the summer.

I probed that lump most of the night, hoping that this greatly enlarged lymph node was my imagination. It just had to be an under-arm muscle I didn't know existed. The lump was accompanied by a searing, stinging pain. I extended my arm under the bright bathroom light and searched for a burn of some sort. Other than the lump, nothing could be seen.

Dr. Stead listened as I described the sensations. She felt the bulging spot. She felt again and again.

"Maybe it is a torn rotator cuff," I offered hopefully. She said nothing.

My thorough doctor felt beneath the other arm. I had done the same myself the night before. Because of the previous mastectomy, a comparison was difficult. Dr. Stead soon detected another enlarged lymph gland, though somewhat smaller than the one on the right.

Feeling my neck like a strangler looking for a good place to grasp, the usually personable doctor robotically remarked that there was a suspicious lymph gland on the left side. Dr. Stead scribbled some notes in the chart. She began discussing treatment options, including a chemotherapy known to be especially hard on the veins.

I stopped her monologue long enough to remind her I was more interested in quality of life than quantity. She listened and politely allowed me finish my point of view. Then she continued as if dying too soon wasn't an option.

"You probably will not lose much hair," she said. That was relief as I finally have my second set of extremely short, but treasured curls.

Dr. Stead continued describing the protocol. My surgically implanted port would be used for administering the drug. She would monitor my blood counts meticulously as they could drop dangerously low. I would come each week for eight weeks and then she would access the progress.

I clearly had two options: continue treatment or "case closed." I thought about the two challenges I had yet to accomplish. One was to publish this journey in a book and the other was to see our son Charlie graduate from college. There are no guarantees regardless of my choice, but my chances are obviously better with treatment.

So here I am, off again on this journey that never seems to end. My cancer may not be cured, but my funny bone will heal soon. I promise.

Journal Entry Forty-Eight

We have a feisty hen named "Mrs. Red" who is sitting. The only problem is that she is not only sitting on her own eggs, but the eggs of all her friends. We have three nests, but all eight of our hens like this special wire one which is where Mrs. Red has decided to sit. We generally get about six eggs a day, for but more than a week we haven't gotten any for cooking. Mrs. Red claims them first. She is presently sitting on over twenty eggs even though I removed a dozen or more when she was off taking parenting class.

Mrs. Red is a funny sight with full wings and out-stretched legs squatting on her maternal throne. I dare not try to take an egg out from under her as she protests loudly and pecks hard. The one time I tried, the rooster came running in full attack armor. Believe me, Mr. Red, with his nine-inch nail spurs, can be most intimidating. You don't mess with his woman.

Now I admit to being a novice chicken farmer, but I never knew hens were so possessive of their eggs. There is no way Mrs. Red can hatch all of those eggs and I am worried about her psychological well-being when she finally realizes this. I made a mistake when I cut class the day my professor taught separation anxiety in Chickenology 101.

I have made many mistakes trying to be a farm girl. Last week I traded several glass paperweights for an antique- looking butter churn. I wanted to make my own butter. I wasn't sure how it was made, but I knew my grandmother used a churn which had a short stick with four wooden prongs on the end. I do have a friend who has a bull, so surely with her knowledgeable guidance, I could make some genuine butter.

After I got my prized churn home and looked more closely at it, I discovered that the handsome bucket didn't look like it had ever been used for making butter. In fact, it was brand-spanking new. I began to be suspicious. Some old-timers who grew up on a farm happened by. I asked them to look at the churn and give me their opinion. Both told me they wouldn't use it for making butter because the small barrel, though nicely detailed, was made of cedar. Come to think of it, the inside of that churn did smell like our cedar chifferobe. Tree-flavored butter wasn't what I had in mind. Instead of a butter churn, we now have a one-of-a-kind, cedar umbrella holder.

When I get past this weekly regimen of chemotherapy and gain back some energy, I do want to try my hand at making home-made mayonnaise and bread. I don't know why I have gotten so interested in domestic doings lately. Buddy will attest that genuine, time-consuming cooking has never been my forte.

As a gift for a special occasion recently, some dear friends gave me money to buy something I especially wanted. It was a toss up between a night at the beach or a new mixer. As much as I love the ocean, the practicality of a new mixer won out. My other one was bought in a yard sale about ten years ago and only ran on high speed. Most criminals do less time for armed robbery than I have spent wiping whipped cream and mashed potatoes off the ceiling and cabinets.

So out with the old mixer and in with the new. Buddy is amused at my new interest in old-time cooking. He believes it will be a short-lived fad. Probably so.

Journal Entry Forty-Nine

This isn't Mother's Day, but I believe everyday should be. Don't ever underestimate the influence of a mama. I *had* one and I *am* one. I can be the most easy-going person in the world unless you mess with my child. Then I am Mrs. Goliath. My mother was the same way. So was her mother.

Whoever said, "The hand that rocks the cradle rules the world," had some worldly wisdom. The influence and love of a mother is like none other.

There is story in the Bible about King Solomon who became known as the wisest man in the world. He was called upon to settle a dispute between two women, each claiming to be the baby's mother. In his wisdom, Solomon pronounced that he would cut the baby in two parts, giving each a half. One woman immediately relinquished her claim. Solomon then knew who the real mother was, the one who was willing to give possession of her baby to another so the child would live.

Though my mother passed away a couple of years ago, there is seldom a day I don't think about her. I know this seems odd, but every time I enter a public restroom stall, I remember Mama. She had this unsolicited, but frequently given advice: "Never go into a restroom stall without tissue in your purse or pocket." She predicted that if you didn't have tissue, there wouldn't be any toilet paper." How right she was about that and many other things.

Mama passed along many other universal truths. One was that you never knew when you were making a life-long memory for your child. Sure enough, Charlie and Bobby remember activities or conversations today that I thought so insignificant at the time. "Mama-prints," is how I think of them now, indelibly etched in the heart of a child.

A friend's cousin had an ordinary mixed-breed dog. She was pregnant. The puppies were due in about ten days. Unfortunately, while running around having a good time in the yard, the riding lawn mower rolled over her small body and both hind legs were completely severed.

The cousin rushed the mutt to the vet who gave her two choices. Sew the gal dog up and allow her to deliver the puppies or put her to sleep. It was an agonizing decision, but the cousin decided she wanted to keep her dog alive.

The veterinarian did a fine job sewing up the gaping holes where the hind legs were. In a matter of days, the dog was walking. She didn't moan and groan. She didn't have a pity party. She didn't worry about whether she could be a good mother. She just accepted her lot in life and adapted the best she could. She would take two steps forward, pull up her backside, take two more steps and pull up her backside again until she finally got where she wanted to go.

That gal dog gave birth to six precious, perfectly healthy puppies. She cleaned them up. She nursed them. She weaned them. And the puppies learned to walk. All of them walked just like her.

Journal Entry Fifty

Some mornings are better than others. At four o'clock a.m. today, I was vomiting, hoping this was my final hasty trip to the bathroom. Not until several hours later was I finally able to climb into bed to stay for a while. This new chemotherapy is meaner than the last one. As predicted, I grow sicker each day while the injected poison does battle with the enemy cancer cells within me.

In a fog of weariness, I picked up the ringing phone by the bedside. It was a friend calling to inform Buddy and me that our mutual friend, Ed Boswell, had passed away.

Ed faithfully read this column. When his eyesight diminished severely because of the diabetes a few months ago, his wife, Joanne, enlarged the type on the computer so he could read the column himself.

Ed had been ill for a long time and his death wasn't a total surprise. Yet, it was still shocking in a way. Even when we know death is coming, the reality of it makes us catch our breath.

Ed clearly recognized me at my last visit. Since Joanne was occupied with a worker from hospice, I sat with Ed, listening mostly, as he talked about whatever came to mind. He flittered from one subject to another, never quite finishing the story he started. Occasionally he would quote bits of recognizable scripture, mostly about heaven.

As it came time to leave, I knew it was unlikely that I would see Ed alive in this world again. My intentional last words to him were, "I love you, Ed. We will see each other again one of these mornings." I leaned over the recliner and gave him a lingering bear hug.

Tears welled in his eyes. In a few seconds, with quivering lips, he said, "I love you, Miss Nancy. You were the best Sunday School teacher I ever had."

This was one of those poignant, memorable moments in life. A huge emotional knot filled my closing throat. Tumultuous tears tumbled down my cheeks. Yes, I was privileged to be Ed and Joanne's Sunday School teacher, but Ed, himself, had taught me so much by example in the years I had known him.

Ed left an impression. He wasn't an elaborate dresser or an elegant speaker. He didn't drive a fancy car. Ed didn't have a lot of money, but if you needed his last dollar, I am sure he would have quickly given it. Ed was a doer, ever eager to give a helping hand to a friend or stranger. Summer before last there was hardly anybody in the county who didn't get a big bunch of his home-grown turnip greens, personally picked and enthusiastically delivered with an unforgettable hearty smile.

Buddy and I first knew Ed and Joanne nearly thirty years ago when we were members of a little country church in Stockbridge, Georgia. For years, Buddy and Ed drove a church bus all around the rural country side picking up boys and girls, bringing them to Sunday School.

Somehow, in my mind's eye of the future, I see all those happy little children rushing around the streets of gold, grabbing hold of his white robe and saying, "Thank you, Mr. Ed. We are here today because of you."

Good-bye for now, Ed, my friend, my brother. See you in the morning.

Journal Entry Fifty-One

For the record, I have postponed taking any more chemotherapy, at least for now. Possibly forever. This was my fifth segment of this regimen of chemotherapy. The second dose of this premeditated poisoning nearly killed me. My obituary came close to reading "death by drowning." I could hardly keep my head above the toilet water.

For the moment I have decided I'd rather die of the disease than the treatment. Except for the dying part, I am ready to go. It is a dilemma really. I don't know whether to make plans or cancel them. While I am waiting around to see if I am going to live or die this round, I thought I would attempt a few interesting projects just to be sure I haven't missed anything.

God really knew what he was doing when he created me during the early 1940's. I could never have made it in the olden days of my grandmother, much less in the days of the pioneers or even further back in the days of manna in the wilderness. Though I try, I cannot seem to master the old ways of doing things.

Take that manna for example. That is a bona fide word straight from the Bible. Manna is bread. God provided it every-day for his people when they were looking for the Promise Land. If I had to depend on my bread-baking abilities to make it to heaven, I wouldn't rise.

Baking sour dough bread was my most recent project. I have a bread machine that makes wonderful bread, but in my humble but accurate opinion, that is cheating. Anybody can dump in the pre-packaged flour and yeast, drop in a tablespoon of tepid water and turn on the switch.

I wanted to make bread the real way. While I didn't major in chemistry or biology, and certainly not Home Economics, I did remember that bread-making involved activating single-celled fungi. The result would cause a wad of flour to expand exponentially.

I went by the directions on the package. Honest. I mixed

the flour, the water and the yeast. I let it sit and grow. Then I beat on that lump and let it sit some more. Each time the arrogant dough came back higher than ever. From Monday until Wednesday, I punched the lump and it did what it was supposed to do. It got puffy. Finally it was time to bake the bread.

The directions on the yeast package said sour dough bread likes humidity. Dutifully I placed a shallow bowl of water in the bottom of the oven. The instructions also said to spray water on the sides of the oven while the bread was baking. Now, *that* was the mistake.

Using the same plastic water bottle that I use on indoor plants, I sprayed the sides of the oven. One squirt. Two squirts. The third squirt ricocheted to the light bulb in the back of the oven. That bulb exploded better than gun powder.

Glass shattered all over the top of the raw dough and just missed my eyes. As I jumped backwards, one bare foot landed on a piece of the broken bulb.

The cut probably needed a half-dozen stitches, but I wasn't about to tell this humiliating tale in the emergency room. I bought these bandage-like doohickeys shaped like butterflies which work just as good as stitches.

They say cats have nine lives. Guess you can call me the "cat lady."

Journal Entry Fifty-Two

I am glad to have the freedom to write occasionally about spiritual matters. Indeed, the spiritual matters.

While in the hospital in 1976, following my third miscarriage, the gynecologist insisted I have a hysterectomy. I emphatically insisted I would not, knowing that I had prayed for years that God would give us a son. I remember the first time I asked God for a son. I was all alone in a thicket of woods behind our home. The sun streamed through the trees. In exchange for this son, I promised that Buddy and I would give him the best Christian up-bringing we could. Also, we would never forget that this boy was a gift on loan from God. We would willingly give this son back to make a difference anywhere in the world.

Walking back to the house in full confidence that God would answer that prayer, I added a motherly postscript. Should God choose to send this coming son of our's down the Amazon River, would He please provide a little row boat so his dad and I could follow behind.

In 1979, the word was that we were again with child. The sonogram confirmed it was a boy. Our friends called us Abraham and Sarah as Buddy was by then no spring rooster. The rhythmical kicking in the womb let me know that there were some music genes in this baby.

By the age of two Charlie was reading. By the age of five, he could play Chariots of Fire on the piano. At the age of twelve, he had his Black Belt in Karate. In eighth grade he was President of the Student Council.

Skip forward a few years. Charlie will soon be a senior at Toccoa Falls College. This is a small, but fully-accredited four-year school in North Georgia.

A couple of weeks ago Charlie told us he wanted to use his brief fall break to go to Philadelphia to work in the homeless shelters. I took a deep breath and said "Okay." Being the most financially insecure one in the family, I asked how much the trip would cost. It was a modest amount. Charlie already had some yard work lined up for the week-end to pay for the trip. No problem.

Then a few days ago Charlie announced the *biggie.* I don't know why it caught us by surprise. We should have been expecting this. While we may temporarily forget a twenty year old prayer, God doesn't. Charlie informed us he would be going to Zambia, Africa, during his winter break in January to do evangelism work in the villages along with a professor and some others.

Practical me. Knowing what a struggle it has been for us to come up with several thousand dollars for tuition each semester, I swallowed hard and cleared my throat a couple of times. Since Charlie had less than $100 in the bank, I casually asked him how he was going to pay the $2300 it would take for travel and other related expenses. He gave me a bewildered look. His response was, "That is God's problem."

My faith wasn't as strong as his that day. "I know, Charlie, but…"

"Mom, raising the money is not my problem. It is not your problem. If God wants me in Africa to work among the native people there, He will provide the way." Case shut.

Charlie got a letter today. I emailed him at the dorm and told him there was an envelope on his mail table formally addressed to Charles E. Kelly. He wrote back and told me to open it since he wouldn't be home for several days. As I opened the letter, my eyeballs broadened and my faith took a quantum leap. In the envelope were three, one-hundred dollars bills with an anonymous note saying to use the money for up-coming trips. Three-hundred dollars. This was exactly what he needed to cover the cost of his passport, his deposit for the Africa trip, and for the inoculations necessary to travel out of the country.

Now, God, about that row boat.

***Addendum**: Every penny needed for the trip came in from several unexpected sources.*

Journal Entry Fifty-Three

It was a dark and rainy night. Dutifully I went outside to check on the goats, chickens, ducks and one lone guinea before calling it a day. The pygmy goats were in the over-sized dog house. A couple of hens and the guinea were high and dry in the barn. The rooster and other hens were roosting in the trees ignoring the drizzle.

The critters were safe. Soaking wet, I hoofed it back into the house. Just a few more chores and I could finally head to bed.

A brief e-mail confirmed that Charlie was back at college. Oppie, our Chihuahua, was under her afghan in the den. Snowball, our recently adopted white cat, was snoozing at the foot of the bed. In the spare bedroom, the thirty-six incubating chicken and guinea eggs were at just the right temperature. All was well with the world. At least I thought so.

I put on my pajamas, downed my medicines and climbed into bed. The last that I remember as I drifted off to sleep was hearing Buddy turning on the shower and the rings on the shower bar curtain being pulled shut.

The telephone by the side of the bed rang. I groped for the phone and struggled to place the proper end to my ear.

"Hello," I answered, trying to sound awake and pleasant.

A gruff voice proceeded. "This is the police. We are in your drive-way. Please go to the door and let us in."

I stumbled down the hall to the front door. I fumbled nervously with the lock. Flashing his badge, one of the officers asked if this was the Kelly household. I answered in the affirmative, fearfully anticipating what was next.

Then it seemed as if a thousand flood lights illuminated the house. The entire front yard was full of happy people carrying balloons. They rushed the porch steps. Leading the crowd was a large man carrying a brightly-colored package.

Buddy gently nudged me back to the edge of the mattress as he climbed into bed himself.

"You were talking in your sleep," he said as he adjusted his pillow, the bedspread and the cat.

"You interrupted my dream," I mumbled. "Now I will never know what was in the package." Buddy didn't have a clue as to what I meant and didn't ask.

I drifted off to sleep again, but the dream never picked up where it left off. I don't remember anything else except the rooster crowing at daybreak.

Journal Entry Fifty-Four

There is an old proverb that says just about anything you want it to. I've been known to make up a couple of mama-isms while raising kids. Like the time one of our foster children choked on a piece of hard candy. In a panic, I turned Bobby up-side down and shook the him by his feet until it popped out. At the tender age of five he probably didn't realize that this bizarre response probably saved his life.

I shudder to think what would have happened to Bobby had he not been removed from a despicable, abusive environment. He entered our home that memorable first day with a tiny teddy bear and a brown grocery sack of quickly-gathered dirty clothes.

Bobby was a winsome child, full of personality. He had a few famous quips of his own. Not long after he became a member of our household, we had some church members for dinner. Bobby loved home-style mashed potatoes which I placed on the table last. He was delighted. An impromptu, but sincere compliment followed: "My mama is the best *mother-cooker* in the whole world." This brought hysterical tears of laughter to our only somewhat righteous table. Unless you grew up in the south, you may not catch the humor. Just be glad for your sheltered up-bringing.

Now an independent young adult, Bobby remembers many of my off-the-cuff adages. He can probably quote this one by heart: "Sometimes life turns you up-side down and you are better off for the experience."

Life is topsy-turvy for us all at one time or another. We learn to deal with it. Sometimes I wonder what my life would have been like if I never had this disease.

For starters, I wouldn't have to schedule my life around doctor appointments and chemotherapy. I wouldn't have to take a dozen pills a day. I wouldn't get those knowing sympathetic looks from others when I walk into a crowded room. I wouldn't need cosmetic support to look esthetically normal. There wouldn't be a portable oxygen tank to wag around or a more permanent one to anchor to at night.

Bobby wouldn't wonder if I'll always be there for him. Charlie wouldn't wonder if I'll be around for his college graduation or his someday marriage. Buddy wouldn't toss and turn, afraid his mate will leave this life before he does. And finally, I wouldn't be writing this journal.

The reality is that I do have cancer. So, if I can only live once, then I must do it right. I purposely put my feet on the floor in the mornings knowing that the clock is ticking down. Strange how many folks long for immortality, yet don't know what to do with themselves on a wet Sunday.

Journal Entry Fifty-Five

Where has a year gone? This time last year I was in the hospital, precariously ill, yet desperately wanting to go home for the holiday. My dance with cancer was going badly and the music was melancholy. Sunnie Anne and Bob, my two youngest siblings, were hastily making their way to Georgia.

This year, if all goes as planned, Buddy, Charlie and I will be enjoying Thanksgiving dinner with the family in Mississippi. I am not well, but neither am I critical. In one word, I am stable. The bone pain is still there, but pain is a good indication that you are still alive.

A lot has transpired in twelve months. My oldest brother Charles had a heart attack while hunting in the woods. Miraculously he survived. My Aunt Carmen in Las Vegas was told she had terminal lung cancer. I am happy to report that she is toughly fighting and has passed her projected expiration date. Survival runs in the family.

The wife of my middle brother, Mike, went through a breast cancer scare. Thankfully the disease was caught early. The young adult son of another sister-in-law had treatment for serious testicular cancer. He, too, is ahead of the game. However, my feisty ninety-eight-year old mother-in-law, never before seriously ill, has become weak, frail and bed-ridden. She wonders why she has lived so long and is eager for the angels to carry her home.

Ironically, both my parents died during Thanksgiving week, sixteen years apart on the same floor of the same hospital in Memphis attended by the same doctor. You might think I dread this time of the year, but I don't. While there are some sad memories, there are many pleasant ones too.

In my closet is a pilgrim dress I frequently wore to Thanksgiving activities when I was a school principal. The bonnet and white apron are yellowing from age, but I never look at that costume without thinking about Tommy.

One of our annual Thanksgiving projects was for all the children to write an essay on thankfulness. The best essays were read in the school assembly. Those who weren't old enough to write essays could draw a picture depicting something for which they were thankful.

While touring a kindergarten room in that pilgrim dress, I noticed Tommy was drawing a realistic-looking turkey: fat body, slender neck, hanging jowls and colorful feathers. When I made a second passing, Tommy was vigorously marking a large black “X” over the turkey. My formal psycho-educational background prodded me. I wondered if Tommy was demonstrating suppressed hostility. I probed for further signs.

"Tommy, that is a lovely drawing of a turkey." He nodded in agreement. "I am puzzled by the big 'X' though. Is this a picture of what you are thankful for?"

Tommy didn't hesitate. "It is. I am thankful that I am *not* a turkey."

Journal Entry Fifty-Six

*J*ust got home from having chemotherapy…not the rough kind that I was previously on, but a kinder one that strengthens the deteriorating bones. There are a few side-effects, but they are tolerable. My doctor gave me prescriptions for no less than thirteen drugs to treat everything from sinus to anemia.

Last Saturday I went to a local health fair. I only went because Buddy wouldn't go unless I did. He skipped the mammogram and I declined the PSA exam. Otherwise, we got the same tests. When the results came back, his blood report was perfect. Not a single component was out of range. He was as euphoric as a child with straight A's on his report card.

I nervously tore open my envelope hoping for equally good news. Alas. Over half of my lab results were flagged as abnormal. When I asked my cancer doctor today what those lab results meant, she answered succinctly, "You are a sick lady."

Hmm. What wisdom.

Lately I have been noticing an enlarged lesion at the end of my spine making it uncomfortable to sit. My oncologist is sending me over the mountain in the morning to see the radiologist. I have had radiation in the sacral area twice. Sinc there are limits to the number of times a body part can radiated, I may get to live the rest of my life standing up.

Cancer is such an inconvenience. I already had plan tomorrow. Lying on a cold x-ray table wasn't one of them. I should have learned Life Lesson #124 better, "Exp unexpected."

One Sunday morning not long ago a restless litt in church with her mother.. "Mommy," she said, "ca now?"

"No" her mother replied. "The preacher is his sermon."

"Well, "she replied, "I think I have to throw up.

The dubious mother responded nonchalantly, "Then go out the front door and around to the back of the church. Throw up behind a bush."

After about sixty seconds, the little girl returned to her seat. "Did you throw up?" the mom asked.

"Yes," the little girl replied.

"How could you have gone all the way behind the church and returned so quickly?"

"I didn't have to go out of the church, Mommy. They have a box next to the front door that says, '*For the Sick*'."

Journal Entry Fifty-Seven

My back side is all marked up with magic markers. I wouldn't chance running naked in the woods just now. A deer hunter might think he had a big one in his scope.

There is a huge "X" on my lower back that an eight-year-old with a BB gun could hit from his second-story bedroom window. That X marks the spot the technicians will shoot with powerful invisible rays tomorrow and several more days thereafter.

I feel discouraged today. Cancer treatment seems ad infinitum and ad nauseum at times. To top it off, there is a three hour round trip to the nearest radiation center. That's what I get for living in the mountains, but the trade-off is worth it.

The computer-driven machines at the cancer treatment center are impersonal. A steady stream of people of all ages and stages of cancer stream in and out of the isolated radiation room. The staff is cordial, but I feel like a prodded cow being forced into the cattle chute. No options except bolting and running away like a soon-to-be altered bull. But I won't kick over the traces. Not today.

Mentally I am prepared. Just smoke me and be done with it. No big deal. Actually it takes longer to undress and dress again than to be zapped. Hopefully the tumor will diminish and the pain will go away for a while.

Eventually this experience will become just another notch on this veteran cowgirl's belt. Maybe I won't succumb to metastasized cancer but of Mad Cow Disease instead.

Journal of a Living Lady

Journal of a Living Lady

. . . continues

Journal Entry Fifty-Eight

I recently experienced a close encounter of the strangest kind. It was late in the afternoon. Relatives were coming for the holidays and I needed a couple of small items from the grocery store. Buddy was snoring in the recliner, so I grabbed the car keys and made a quiet exit. I would be back in a jiffy, provided the creek didn't rise or a night stalker didn't choose me for his prey.

I stopped at one of our community's locally-owned markets. The chain grocery store was ten miles away and the minor savings wouldn't be worth the gas. A cold blast of wind whipped the hat from my head. I grabbed it on the fly as I hustled through the front door of the little grocery.

A dark-haired young man was finishing up his purchase at the cash register. I greeted him and the cashier with a nod and made my way to the bread aisle. Moments later a male voice startled me. "Are you the lady I see in the newspaper?"

I turned around for a better look. It was the same man I had passed coming into the store. His ruddy face looked wind-blown.

"Yes, I write for the paper," I replied, puzzled by the unexpected interruption.

The lanky man, probably in his late thirties, extended a loose, wristy handshake while mumbling an introduction. I didn't recognize the name or the face.

It was then I got a whiff of his alcoholic breath. If somebody had lit a match to the fumes, the whole place would have exploded. This guy was beyond tipsy.

He studied my face for a couple of seconds. "You ain't nearly as ugly as people say you are." He paused briefly. "But you are a good person. I know that."

"Thank you," I murmured, not knowing what else to say to the uncouth stranger. I had a feeling this wasn't going to be a routine encounter with a loyal reader.

" I am a Yankee," the man volunteered. He continued without hesitation. "I love you."

My adrenal glands signaled for flight. "Thank you," I replied. My mind raced into over-drive as I tried to determine how to quickly and quietly exit the store without causing a commotion.

The man made a move toward me. He came so close that his nose almost collided with mine. I recoiled thinking he was going to *kiss* me.

"Now that we are in love with each other..." he whispered.

For a second I lost my breath. Then I backed away and nervously laughed, wondering what the rest of that sentence might be. I'll never know.

"Nice meeting you," I said as I hastened down the aisle abruptly. Out of the corner of my eye, I saw the fellow hesitate briefly and then leave through the front door. Through the large store window, I watched the man stagger across the parking lot. He crossed the busy highway and continued up the hill.

I have no clue where he came from or where he was going. But, rest assured that the next time I need a few items from the market, I'll take the recliner and send Buddy to the quick pick up store.

Journal Entry Fifty-Nine

*O*kay. This is a new year and time to take the annual reality check which is slightly more fun than the annual procto check.

Realty #1: I am living daily in the final two minutes of the game I think. Then again, I have been told *that* and thinking that for over two years now. Other than a for a few cliff-hanging set-backs, I have continued to function fairly normally. This just proves that God likes to dumbfound the medical statisticians.

Reality #2: I am still fat. While I did go through a phase of dropping several pounds, I am almost back at my set-point. Guess I have done too much sitting and pointing. Even cancer hasn't been successful in making me lean enough to shop for a size ten. If cancer would guarantee rapid weight loss, I am certain there would be some people who would stand in line to buy it.

Reality #3: Buddy is never going to change. After all these years you would think I could have reformed him by now. I give up. He is always going to clear his throat while talking on the telephone, start eating before I have finished cooking the bread and continue taking out only *part* of the trash. This husband of mine annoyingly reminds me to wash my hands after being out in public. He will check my oxygen tanks several times a day to be sure I have enough in reserve. He will never cease to ask me daily if I have taken my vitamins or aspirin and, though he startles me at times, he will keep kissing me gently when my eyes are closed.

Reality #4: I am blessed.

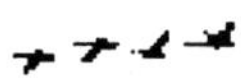

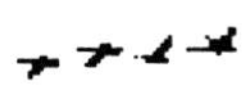

Journal Entry Sixty

The holidays were nice. I got a reprieve from chemotherapy and radiation. I didn't have to check in with the doctor even once. But, alas, it is back to the real world. More chemo today. As usual the doctor's office was packed. Some of us were tucked into small rooms to receive our I. V. drips. Others were pricked for blood. Appointments were scheduled for next week, next month, whenever.

The cancer-war saga continues with new recruits daily. Four of my friends joined the battle just in the last month. Lung cancer. Colon cancer. Breast cancer. Bladder cancer.

We veterans think of cancer in colors. Green light…the cancer is active. Red light…the cancer is cured or at least in remission. Yellow light…somewhere in between.

Yellow. That's my color right now. First it was green. Then red light for 12 years. Then green for two and now yellow.

I have never been a fan of the color yellow. It looks yucky on me. I used to have such rosy cheeks that my own mother accused me wearing rouge. Now my hemoglobin stays so low I take shots and drink red Kool-Aid.

Aging and cancer have taken their toll on me for sure. My mind doesn't only wander, it completely leaves me sometimes. Guess creeping senility is one reason why God doesn't allow most women over 50 to have babies. They would put them down somewhere and forget where they put them.

My doctor tells me to stay in touch with my body. Frankly mine isn't all that communicative. I did hear from it on one of my good days lately when I said, "Body, how about us trying some good old-fashioned exercise."

Clear as a bell my yellow body called out, "Crazy woman. Get over it!"

Journal of a Living Lady

. . . continues

Journal Entry Sixty-One

When the phone rings at two in the morning, it can't be good news. It wasn't. Buddy's mother had just died. Actually it was a blessing. Maggie Clytee Kelly was ninety-eight years-old and had been ready to move on for a long time. "I don't know why we old folks live so long," she would frequently say.

Mother K. was a tall, big-boned woman whose black hair turned a gorgeous silver during my marriage to Buddy. Until last year, she had never been an in-patient in the hospital or been seriously ill. She didn't drink or smoke, but ate fried chicken, pork chops, eggs and anything else she wanted. When Mother Kelly came to visit us in Atlanta, there was always a mandatory trip to the mall for a singular purpose: to get one of Truett Cathy's famous Chick-fil-A sandwiches.

For many years Mother Kelly lived in an unpretentious three-room frame house on the main drag through town. She had a high school diploma, uncommon for that early era, as well as a life-time teaching certificate. During her later working years, she made her livelihood by sewing.

Mother K. had a sense of humor that endeared her to me from that first time we met. I was just nineteen when Buddy drove me from Memphis to the little town of Boyle, Mississippi, to meet my future mother-in-law. In the course of our getting acquainted, I admitted to not knowing how to hem pants. She immediately sat me down to teach me how. I was all thumbs and repeatedly pricked her with the sewing needle, sometimes drawing blood. She mocked like a howling dog each time I stabbed her, causing me to laugh like a hysterical hyena. To this day I still can't hem pants properly. If Buddy needs something hemmed, I use contact glue and scotch tape.

Buddy would tell you Maggie Clytee was a wonderful mother not only to him, but to his older brother, Thomas and only sister, Ann, who came much later in life. When Buddy's father died in a wreck, Mother K. raised Ann as a single mother. She did a fine job rearing all three of her children. I will always be grateful for the up-bringing she gave Buddy. He has her good, practical qualities.

Mother Kelly was a Christian through and through. She taught Sunday School most of her life and could quote Scripture at the drop of a hat. It is said that many men marry women like their mothers. I doubt I could ever live up to Mother Kelly. She was a jewel. Ironically, she died on my own mother's birthday.

Journal Entry Sixty-Two

The chronic dropsies. That is what I call it. In the past week, at different meals, I have deposited food in the middle of the kitchen floor. First it was a bowl of home-cooked spaghetti. Then it was a plate of fried okra and finally a tray of baked potato skins. If the linoleum had been spotless enough, we might have reclined like the ancients and feasted with our fingers. Unfortunately it wasn't. This didn't keep Oppie, our Chihuahua, and Snowball, our cat, from declaring the food theirs. It was a chore for Buddy and me to keep them away as we scooped up the mess into the dust pan along with shards of shattered glass.

My strength has been ebbing little by little. Buddy whispers to all our friends, as if I don't see him, that my color is off. He hasn't fussed a bit over the lost food though I tend to think it is my klutziness instead of weakness. He just cleans up and tells me it is no big deal.

I finally gave in and made an appointment with my doctor. He immediately sent me to the hospital for a transfusion. I expected so.

It was a disappointment that my designated donor couldn't provide blood for me. I have known this guy since the day he was born. I know he exercises regularly and normally eats right. Grilled meat. No mayo. Water to drink. To my knowledge he has never touched drugs or alcohol and isn't a smoker. What an ideal donor. He even has my blood type, Rh A negative, not extremely rare, but not common either. Charlie gives blood regularly anyway. Why not to me, his mother?

Seems that there are other factors involved. Something called antibodies that may or may not match even if the type does. Another deterrent was that he just recently returned from Africa and might have picked up something *his* healthy immune system could handle, but not my impaired one. Bottom line. I had to have a stranger's blood.

As always, there was a mountain of paperwork to complete. Checks and double checks. The strangest form was the one that made me acknowledge in writing that nothing could replace blood. I sort of knew that anyway. Even the ancient scriptures say that *the life of the flesh is in the blood.* While that inspired statement has theological implications, it has practical ones too.

As the infusion trickled into my veins, I fanned Buddy to keep him from fainting. Quietly I wondered who supplied this blood for my benefit. Was he or she a pillar of society or a homeless human being? Was he Republican or Democrat? Was he of Christian belief or not? Was he black or white? It didn't matter. Precious crimson blood shows no prejudice or partiality.

Thank you, donor, whomever you are.

Journal Entry Sixty-Three

*T*his morning Buddy ran into the house in a panic wanting me to call the veterinarian. He sounded like Prissy in *Gone with the Wind*, "Lawdsy, we've got to have a doctor! I don't know nothing abôut birthing babies."

We have had two pygmy goats since last June. One was a young billy and the other an unproven nanny. Both got very fat on the summer grass and generous feed. We might have suspect-ed Cola was expecting except that Pistol was just as fat. Yet, when Cola's bag dropped a few days ago, we were fairly confident of an impending delivery. We just wished it didn't have to be February, one the coldest months of the year.

Today Cola started bellowing. No, that is what cows do. She started baaing. No that is what sheep do. Whatever, she was hollering in goat language. Labor no doubt. Been there, done that. It ain't fun.

"Call the vet and see what we need to do," Buddy said. I reminded him that animals had been giving birth for many centuries without veterinarian assistance. To ease his mind, I went out to the barn to see if Cola was truly in distress. She wasn't.

First came a black kid about the size of our Chihuahua. The second kid was the caramel color of both registered parents. Yes, Bristol Pistol, the head of the goat family, and NiCola had to register. That way goat genealogists can trace their family tree just like the Aristocratic King Canines do.

Buddy had seen calves born. I have raised exotic birds and worms. Goats were new to both of us, especially *registered* goats.

Coincidentally, our son Charlie was home from college in time to observe the kidding. I was glad. Maybe he would have empathy when his someday future wife was delivering our first grandchild.

In comparison to Charlie's arrival, NiCola's birthing was remarkably easy. In less than twenty minutes NiCola had two kids, a boy and a girl. It took twenty hours to have Charlie. Then it was by Caesarean. The obstetrician did a fine job without Buddy's assistance.

After months of mock labor practice, this only father in the Lamaze class with graying hair couldn't bring himself to watch the delivery of our son. It was just as well. Buddy would have fainted anyway. I am certain of it. In his haste to get me to the hospital, he brushed his teeth with hemorrhoid ointment. He denies it, but I was there.

So, here we are twenty-one years later, older and wiser and still able to laugh at ourselves. There is nothing like kidding. Goat kidding that is. In the bathtub are our two baby goats wrapped in pink and blue blankets.

St. Jude Children's Research Hospital

ALSAC • Danny Thomas, Founder

Finding cures. Saving children.

stjude.org

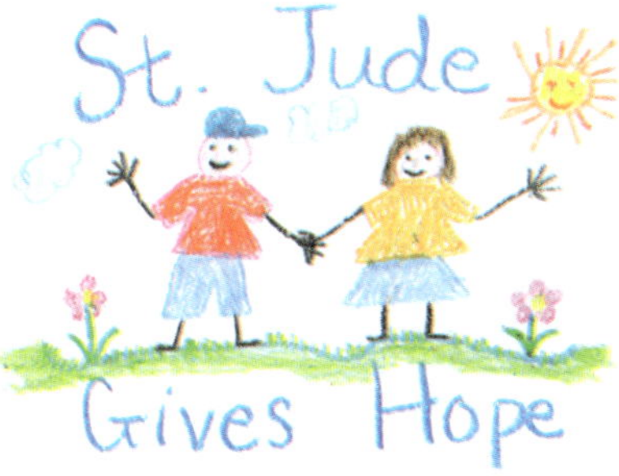

Journal Entry Sixty Four

Charlie is twenty-one today. This column is dedicated to him. Happy Birthday, son.

With the recurring cancer, I never thought I'd live to see the day you reached true adulthood. I think a few doctors are surprised too. How thankful I am for the fine young man you are. I would not trade you for a thousand other sons or a zillion dollars. I would give my life for you in a heart beat. That is how most mothers are, but I feel blessed beyond measure. Let me tell you why.

Even though your dad and I wanted a large family, it was evident early in our marriage that this was unlikely. After three miscarriages spanning several years, we were discouraged. Yet, we were somewhat able to fill that emptiness by raising other people's children. Foster parenting was rewarding, but definitely not easy. Each time one of those children left, sometimes after years in our care, my fractured heart ached so deeply I thought I would literally die.

Though Dad and I didn't see it at the time, all twelve of those children who came through our home were part of God's plan, both for them and for us. Still, we longed for a child of our very own.

I remember one specific day going to a spot in the woods where the sunlight boldly shone through the tree tops as if a beam straight from heaven. I literally begged the Lord to give us a son who would be flesh of our flesh, bone of our bone. Faith is not believing God can. It is believing that he will. I believed with every ounce of my being that God would give us that son.

In the fall of 1979, very early in your gestation, I had a scary experience. The pregnancy test clearly indicated we were expecting. The doctor said we were going to have a baby. But, after a mini-miscarriage crisis, I just had to be sure you were still alive.

I read in the morning paper that there was a clinic in

Atlanta that was giving free pregnancy tests and sonograms. Dad went to work and, unknowing to him, I drove downtown.

Several young teens huddled in the crowded waiting room. Some girls had boyfriends, but most were alone. After reading a couple of magazines, a nurse escorted me to a tiny examining room and instructed me to undress. She left the door slightly ajar. Through the hallway I watched a haggardly-looking doctor hastily checking patients behind make-shift curtains. Eerie moans stirred my curiosity. Before I had time to reflect on the strange scenario, the nurse reappeared and squeezed some cold, gooey gel on my stomach.

"Is this your first baby?" she asked.

"Yes," I replied, not wishing to explain further. She quietly moved the small disc around my belly and listened with a stethoscope. In a few seconds she announced that she had found your heart beat. I was ecstatic. I could see your tiny heart pulsating on a video screen.

"How far along am I?"

The nurse removed a tiny calculator and ruler from the pocket of her smock. "About sixteen weeks," she replied. "When do you want to have your abortion?"

I shot up from that cold metal table clutching the white paper drape tightly to my body. The fiercest tigers of India could not have pulled it away from me.

"Abortion!" Is that what this is, an abortion clinic?"

The nurse looked puzzled. "Of course. Didn't you know?"

"No, I didn't know." I grabbed my clothes from the wall hook. My voice quivered with emotion. "That doctor in there will be doing hysterectomies on Brahma bulls before this baby ends up in the bucket of a butcher parlor."

The stunned nurse turned toward the door and gave a sigh of relief. "That is the most refreshing thing I have heard all day."

So, Charlie, you escaped being an abortion victim that day. Very soon afterwards I was happily wearing maternity clothes. Excitement filled our home and our community. Your dad was a strutting 48 year-old arthritic rooster. Our church friends teasingly called us Abraham and Sarah.

Even today strangers often assume you are our grandson. Well, in a way they are right. You are a grand son, Charlie, all that Dad and I had hoped and prayed you would become.

We don't know what lies ahead for you now, son. Dad and I have done our job. We have loved you, educated you and have tried to impart some important values in the process.

Today you set sail on the sea of adult life. Let the Bible be your compass. We are confident that our God, your God, will continue to direct your journey.

Happy Birthday, our man-child, and Bon Voyage.

Love always,

Mom

Journal of a Living Lady

. . . continues

Journal Entry Sixty-Five

Buddy is not a connoisseur of elegant words. He is poetically challenged. Trust me when I say Buddy doesn't know a sonnet from a sun bonnet. Finishing an elementary *Roses are Red* verse would be a formidable task for him. There is an explanation for his lack of rhyming aptitude.

Keeping food on the table took priority over education in the depression era. Yet, Buddy did finish high school and later the Embry-Riddle School of Aviation much to his credit. Though a poor poet, he is a great aircraft mechanic and a mighty fine husband.

Buddy grew up working Mississippi fields with stubborn mules. He didn't read poetry while pushing a plow or relax under a willow tree penning his inner thoughts. A practical fellow, my Buddy is. He is sentimental, but never gushy.

Imagine my surprise when I opened the daily newspaper yesterday and found an envelope addressed to "Nannio." Nobody calls me that but Buddy. It is his pet name for me, used only and always as a name of endearment.

While not a poet, Buddy is artistic. The envelope was hand-decorated with colorful hearts, arrows and frilly little swirls. This is a departure from his usual doodling of horse derrieres and swishing tails.

I gently pulled at the glued edges of the paper envelope, not wanting to spoil Buddy's unusual canvas. Inside was a note that began, *"In my heart I wonder why it so often seems to be I can never say the things that really mean the most to me."*

Each line was beautifully crafted with such depth of emotion. Buddy appended the poem with carefully underlined words, *"<u>You are so beautiful to me</u>!"* He tediously embellished the bottom corner of the page with an exploding red heart.

I take it all back. Maybe Buddy is a poet after all, a brilliant one at that. Then, perhaps not. In fact, I seriously doubt it. His neat signature hints plagiarism:

Henry Wadsworth Kelly

Journal Entry Sixty-Six

I have accumulated stacks of those "patient copy" sheets. The doctor's receptionist handed me another one as I was about to leave the office. Usually I glance at the balance and then stick it in my purse. Eventually I will get a genuine bill after the insurance company has determined how little they will pay. I used to gasp at balances in the thousands of dollars. Now I am so accustomed to seeing those big figures that they seem ho-hum.

"Can't get blood out of a turnip," my mama used to say. Buddy and I pay what we can. So far we have survived. We continue to have our house and some food in the refrigerator. The car is in the driveway and Charlie is still in college.

This time it wasn't only the balance on the pink form that grabbed my attention. It was all the weird numbers listed under the diagnosis category. Why can't a doctor just write in plain English what is wrong with a patient? How do you interpret such secret codes as: 174.4, 198.5, 197.0, 284.8, and 518.83?

Curiosity got the best of me. I added up all the numbers and they came to a total of 1,373.53. A number that large must mean I am mighty sick, probably nigh unto death. I wasn't too surprised since I have known for a while that I have terminal cancer. Even spent a few months in hospice, but decided I wasn't ready to check out on life in six months or less.

After a little sleuthing on the Internet, I discovered that these numerical digits are called ICD-9 codes. They are cryptic short-hand numbers used for filing insurance claims. Those mystic diagnostic codes probably serve an even nobler secondary purpose: preventing coronaries on the spot.

It is with selfish interest that I reveal to you readers the official interpretation of my own ICD-9 codes. Surely you will want to bring the family food. At the very least, go ahead and decide on a floral arrangement for my imminent demise.

Now, for those of you who are dying to know, these are

the numbers straight from the pink form I got last week.

Warning: these descriptions are not for the weak-hearted. Pregnant women should stop now. Go to the store for pickles or something

NANCY LEE WHITE KELLY

174.4	Breast cancer; malignant neoplasm
198.5	Secondary bone cancer
197.0	Cancer metastasis to the lung
284.4	Aplastic anemia due to systemic disease
518.83	Chronic respiratory failure

I approve the use of diagnostic codes. No physician in their right mind would write all this out for a patient to read casually on the way to the car.

If my Buddy were to ever read such a list about himself, I assure you he would promptly quit breathing. All the CPR skill in the medical world could not revive him..

No denial here. I accept the fact that I am seriously sick. However, I still plan on living forever. So far so good.

Journal Entry Sixty-Seven

Buddy snored heavily, interrupting my brief sleep and diverting my anxious dreams. This would be the night. The odds were greatly against it. I even had doubts myself.

My eyes glanced at the jerky writing on the note that lay on the lighted night stand. It was signed WOULD-BE QUEEN. God, please let it happen.

Vowed and determined to accomplish this one task, I was off on my secret mission. Come swell or high water, rain, sleet or snow, nothing was going to keep me from doing this act of kindness. If I didn't make it back alive, well…so be it. It's been a good life.

I was going among the living, well the semi-living. I consider nursing homes to be way-stations between earth and eternity. I have seen the best of them and probably some of the worst. Me, when my time comes, I prefer a straight ticket without the stop-over.

It was a long drive to this quasi-rest home. I can't tell you where or even the when. Not even the who. But I'll call her Mrs. Peacock. It was a night Mrs. Peacock and the living lady will not likely forget.

I get lots of mail. Not surprising some of my most loyal readers are lonely, little ole ladies as well as a few senior gents. Many are stuck away and abandoned by loved ones. You know how busy life gets. I consider these grand friends *very* special.

I turned off the car lights and eased my vehicle into the parking lot of a run-down old brick building. Happy Acres. That is what Mrs. Peacock sarcastically calls the place in her barely legible hand-printed letters.

I watched the emptiness of the long hallway. Finally I caught a glimpse of a singular worker carrying a cup of coffee. Gently closing the car door, I inched my way to the rear of the building. A broken concrete block in the doorway allowed some fresh night air into the malodorous hall.

I dashed to an idle wheelchair in an alcove. A forgotten afghan became a cloak for my head and shoulders. Fortunately, right across the hall was Mrs. Peacock's room. At least the name plate said so. The door was fully opened. I observed the old woman toss and turn When the coast was clear, I slipped into her room and sat in the straight chair beside her bed.

"Mrs. Peacock," I whispered. "It's me. I told you I would come."

Startled at first, she stretched out her frail hand and felt my face. "I just knewed you would," she said. There was happiness in her voice.

"Is the Midnight Queen up for a little ride?" I asked.

"I am if you are," she said as she sat up on the bed. I helped her put on a robe and some slippers.

"We won't get in trouble, will we?" I asked.

"Who they gonna call?" Mrs. Peacock feebly asked. "Ain't nobody gonna miss me."

She was a consenting adult and was at Happy Acres on her own free will. Still I doubted they would approve such an unorthodox adventure. We snuck out the back door like mischievous school kids. I held onto her tightly, looking over my shoulder to be sure nobody was the wiser. Mrs. Peacock was escaping, albeit temporarily. This had been her fantasy. I was glad to be a part of it.

We drove a mile or two to a rustling stream and sat for a long time. We watched the moon and pretended to see trout jumping between the rocks. We laughed at silly knock-knock jokes. I gave her some party games to play with the old folks at Happy Acres: **Spin the Mylanta Bottle.* * *Red Rover, Red Rover, the Nurse says Bend Over.* * *Twenty Questions Shouted into your Good Ear.*

Mrs. Peacock laughed so hard I could smell urine. It was time to take her back.

In her room at Happy Acres, Mrs. Peacock settled down

on the edge of the bed. In my coat pocket was a gift I slowly unfurled. Mustering my most magical voice I quietly announced, "Mrs. Leona Peacock, I hereby crown you Queen for the Night." Then I carefully placed a golden cardboard crown on top of her wiry-white hair.

Mrs. Peacock removed the crown. Tears welled in her worn eyes as she gazed at the crown in disbelief. Her bony fingers felt around the diamond-shaped ridges.

"Put it on that shelf," she said, pointing to a rack in front of her metal bed. "That way I will always know that this weren't a dream."

Somewhere in Somewhereville in an old rest home is a golden Burger King crown sitting on a rusty-gray shelf. Proof that dreams do come true, even for the aged, if you only believe.

Night. Night.

Journal of a Living Lady

. . . ✍ ends

With renewed strength, I shall continue my trek tomorrow. The most important thing I have learned in this journey is to never put a period where God has placed a comma.

BOOK ORDER FORM

Journal of a Living Lady

Name:____________________________________

Library/Bookstore:______________________________

Street:____________________________________

P.O. Box:_________________________________

City:______________________________________

State:_____ Zip:_____________

Phone:( )____________ Fax: ( )______________

Enclosed is: $14.95 for each book, plus $3.00 s/h for first book. Add $2 each for additional copies.

#Books____ X $14.95 + (s/h)______ = $_________ **Total Enc.**

Georgia residents should add 7% sales tax.

Mail order to:

Kelly Publications

P.O. Box 285

Young Harris, GA 30582

Phone: 706-379-1085 / 379-1488

Fax: 706-379-4123

e-mail: kellypub@alltel.net -or-

kellypublications@hotmail.com